About the Author

Uwe Albrecht was born in Germany in 1966 and is a physician and pioneer of energy medicine. In addition to conventional medicine, he studied traditional Chinese medicine (TCM), classical European healing methods, physioenergetics, osteopathic repositioning techniques (AORT), homeopathy, holistic biological medicine, emotional therapies and sacred geometry. Based on his findings, experiences and insights, Uwe developed *innerwise*®, an energy healing system. For more information visit: *www.innerwise.com*.

Other English books by Uwe Albrecht:
Innerwise®: *The Complete Healing System*
(Card deck with instructional booklet)

Yes/No: Using the Arm-Length Test for Instant Answers and Wellbeing

innerwise®: *Healing All That Lives*

The Imago Game

A Course in Healing

Energy Medicine for Everyone

by

Uwe Albrecht, MD

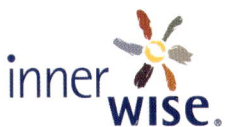

Translated to English by Angelika Hansen.
Edited by Irina Pálffy-Daun-Seiler
with assistance of Tara Rose Gladstone

Disclaimer

The information presented in this work is in no way intended as medical advice or as a substitute for medical treatment. This information should be used in conjunctionwith guidance and care of your physicion, especially if you are taking medications. This book is sold with the understanding that the publisher and the author are not liable for the misconception or misuse of the information provided. Every effort has been made to make this book as complete and accurate as possible. The sole purpose is to educate. The author and publisher shall have neither liability nor responsibility to any person or entity with respect to any loss, damage, or injury caused or alleged to be caused directly or indirectly by the information contained in this book.

Copyright © 2014 Waterfront Digital Press
Text copyright © 2014 Uwe Albrecht

All Rights Reserved.
No part of this publication may be reproduced or transmitted in any form or by any means, electronic or mechanical, including photocopy, recording or any other information storage and retrieval system, without the prior agreement and written permission of the publisher except in case of quotations embodied in critical articles and reviews.
For information, contact *info@innerwise.eu*

Printed in China

Published by Waterfront Digital Press
Cardiff California USA

Graphic by Anna Badowska, Silke Kröger,
Katharina Kosak, Eric Frank
Photos by Hannah Albrecht, Birgit Frank
Text design Keller&Keller GbR Germany
Cover design Rootz&Wingz

First Edition.

ISBN-13: 978-1-941768-04-4

To all my wonderful children:

Jakob (the honest one)
Jonas (the natural one)
Hannah (the shining one)
Luca (the bold one)
Gaia (the one who sees)
Shanti (the courageous one)
Pablo Odin (so eager for life)
Cuinn Bela (the long awaited)

Content

Energy medicine for everyone   ix

1. Why do our lives often not proceed the way we want them to?   1
2. Life energy—the magic power   7
3. The arm-length test—talk with your subconscious   12
4. Do people who are ill want to be ill?   29
5. Journey through the rhythms of our body   37
6. Do we get sick from viruses or bacteria?   42
7. Let's try saying "thank you!"   48
8. I am your symptom   59
9. *innerwise*®: *The Complete Healing System* Self-treatment for everyone   65
10. The bigger picture   79
11. The best sleeper be their king   86
12. Does eating make me ill?   96
13. How do I communicate honestly?   104
14. A relationship or love—that is the question   112
15. Mine—Yours—Ours: The problems we share   127
16. Basic training: How to become an environmental toxicologist   132
17. Who am I, and how many?   138
18. Healing the "soul pie"   148
19. Do I tolerate my dental materials, vitamins and medications?   154

20. The divine stockpot   162
21. Healing the past   167
22. Let he who is without sin cast the first stone . . .   177
23. The big clean-up: first your home, then your life   183
24. Yes to love!   189
25. Yes to the 195   195
26. Finally happy!   202
27. When you're in the flow, success is inevitable   210
28. The Great Mother   216
29. Your personal Independence Day   226
30. Declaring love to Mr. Mind, your conscious brain   231

Epilog   238

Biography of Uwe Albrecht   240

Annex:

Emergency help in case of blockages   246 — Your daily health check   246 — Your weekly health check   247 — Your success check   248 — Make a wish   249 — How high is your level of life energy?   249 — Calculation formula   249 — The moment of truth   250 — The self-denial test   250 — Be a private detective and identify your troubles   251 — Quit the game   252 — Test your biological age in years   252 — The "non-lovable" list   253

Bibliography   254

ENERGY MEDICINE
FOR EVERYONE

Energy medicine is the healing art of the 21st century.

With A *Course in Healing*, everyone can learn and expand on it.

In a humorous way, protagonists *Mr. Mind* and *Mrs. Heart* will guide you through the different topics.

And *The Doc* enriches the experience with his medical knowledge and background. With the help of various practical exercises for self-application at every step, you'll become familiar with energy medicine, healing yourself and your environment, and start to feel safe using it.

Additional meditations and videos for many of the exercises can be experienced through *www.a-course-in-healing.com*.

Become your own healer and find your energy, your freedom and your happiness!

Since the beginning of time, humanity has been familiar with energy healing methods; and although the manifestation of them is diverse in different cultures, ultimately, their core is identical.

They all make the connections and patterns beyond the surface visible, let us discover profound truths and have the capacity to bring you back into the flow of life on all levels of your Being. Energy medicine doesn't eliminate symptoms; it eliminates the causes of them. Then, the symptoms disappear by themselves.

Why aren't all human beings healthy, beautiful, sexy and successful? They all want to be, don't they?

And who really has a say in our lives? Is it our mind, our will, or unconscious forces like our subconscious? It isn't Mr. Mind, our will. He has only acquired 5% of the shares in life decisions, though he considers himself capable of compensating the rest with his big mouth.

Our subconscious owns the other 95%, which shows us clearly with whom we *really* have to talk!

This is the reason why people who are ill stay ill, people who are unsuccessful stay unsuccessful and those who are unhappy stay unhappy. Their subconscious wants it that way. And this is not because of wickedness, but because there is something to be learned or cleared up. The subconscious simply wants to help us act like grown-ups and assume responsibility for our lives. We've created everything in our lives ourselves, and therefore we're the only ones who can change it. Our subconscious reminds us of this fact, which is really rather nice of it, don't you think?

With *A Course in Healing* you learn to communicate with your subconscious, to understand it and to change its programs. You change its energetic charges with the help of energy medicine. Then, people who are ill can become healthy, unsuccessful people can become successful and unhappy people can become happy; and all of this without any help from outside.

This is a course that gives us freedom!

In our lives, we all are on a dance floor moving to the music that fills the room. Very often this music is not our own music, but a mixture of distorted sounds from unresolved situations in our lives.

The simplest way to dance differently, more freely, more beautifully and to one's own rhythm is to change the music.

And energy healing methods do exactly that; they change the music, and then reality follows almost automatically.

I'm a physician, and for 18 years I've been practicing exclusively energy medicine. This means that I've treated all my patients' illnesses and problems in this manner. No painkillers, no antibiotics, no blood pressure pills and no Viagra. In addition to conventional medicine, I also studied the healing arts of many cultures and searched for their congruent essence, which I found with the help of my true teachers—my numerous patients. I've adapted what I've learned in such a way that anyone can easily apply it to his or her own healing process.

I hope that you have great fun with *A Course in Healing*—I sure did.

Uwe Albrecht

The Players

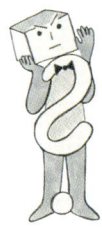

Mr. Mind

Is a minority shareholder and very moody. He thinks he's extremely important, however, in reality he has no power to decide anything. He is our conscious mind.

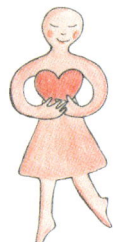

Mrs. Heart

The great *éminence grise* (the grey or invisible eminence). She is our feelings, our subconscious and the one with the *real* power.

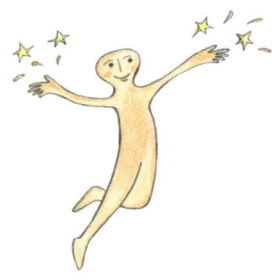

This is you

You have also been given role because you're the protagonist in this course in healing.

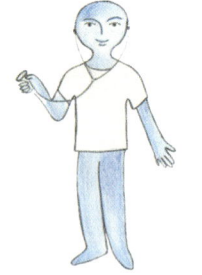

The Doc

This is me—Uwe, with my experiences as a human being, medical doctor, father and mentor.

1.

WHY DO OUR LIVES OFTEN NOT PROCEED THE WAY WE WANT THEM TO?

*I am important.
I am beautiful.*
*I am sexy.
I am successful.
I have the power to achieve anything I want.*

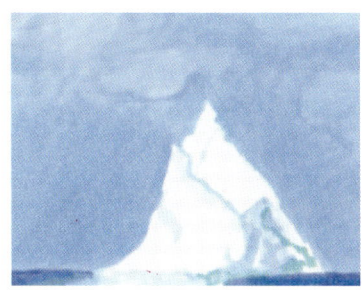

Yeah right! Dream on.

And who are you?!?

Look down for a moment.
I am the part of our iceberg that lies beneath the surface, you little mound.

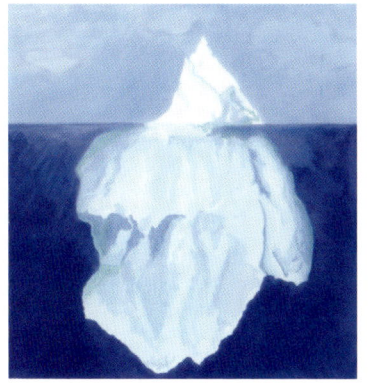

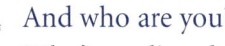
And who are you?
Who's reading these words right now?
You will probably say:
I'm me. I'm . . . (your first name).

Though in reality, there's only a small chance that you're you. This is usually only true for one out of four people. The stability of our identity is the grand illusion of our lives.

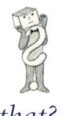 *What are you saying, Doc? How come you know, and who are you anyhow to be suggesting something like that?*

I am just a good practitioner and observer who enjoys thinking for himself. Here's an example for why I may say something like that:

A friend of mine came to me for a treatment. I asked him to say: "I am I." He did indeed say it, but the arm-length test, our lie detector that allows us to talk directly to our subconscious said "no."

I told my friend: "Say it again and use your first name," which he did. "I am Robert," and again the arm-length test said "no." This means: "He is lying."

Then I asked him to say: "I am Franziska"—the name of his wife. Now the lie detector said "yes."

What a mess: There before me was this 220-pound man, and his subconscious asserted seriously that he was his wife.

Don't worry, he was not crazier than three quarters of humanity who have problems with their identity, and it's not little green pills he needs in order to feel happy.

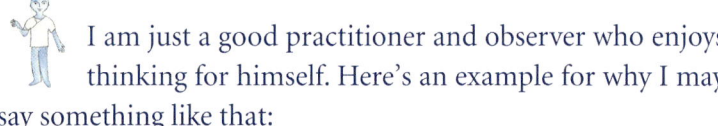 *Hey Doc, what do you mean talking about a lie detector? What kind of esoteric nonsense is that anyway? Something like a pendulum? I am the master of the voice, so with whom are you talking using the arms? Not with me, that's for sure!*

Let me explain this to you big mouth.

I'm your inner wisdom, your subconscious and your emotion; simply put, I'm your heart. You have only acquired about one to five percent of the shares of our mutual iceberg, because you believed that you're sitting on top of it anyway, and you have the power over the voice and parts of the brain.

But have you ever tried to control the smell of a fart? Or to achieve an orgasm by using only your thoughts? To heal an illness or to feel love with your will?

You have no choice but to accept that I—the subconscious—exist. With about 95 to 99 percent of the shares that I hold, you're not even invited to the shareholders' meetings when decisions are made.

Which also means you don't have that much control over a human being and his or her life. And that includes the arms' length, baby.

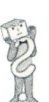 *But look here; I can flex muscles.*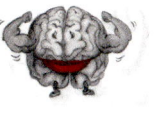
See how strong I am?
Are you trembling with fear now, you little pip-squeak?

 Just because you control the voice doesn't mean that everything you've got to say is of importance. You heard me perfectly well; almost everything in life is defined by me. I create all profound and effective programs and patterns.

Now you'll probably ask yourself: Why is that?

Very simple: I see to it that human beings learn something while here on Earth; that they can experience things and attain wisdom.

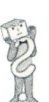 *But that's something I can do as well.*

Sorry to say, but you suffer from the insignificant-little-man syndrome, and you lack the heart—you're just gumption on short legs. But the most important thing to be aware of is that you're in a negative mood most of the time. One negative thought after the other. You're mainly consumed by fear. If you really—heaven forbid—had the power to get your point across, humanity would have long ago erased itself.

I'm rapidly losing interest in continuing in this way with you. It seems that I am the idiot and the bogeyman in this book, the Omega. That's not fair, I don't deserve to be treated like that. I am smart. I've had it; I'm leaving!

Sure, why don't you try? The tip of the iceberg wants its independence. You know, the funniest part is that if you break off, a big part of you will go down and become part of me.

A reincarnation of Mrs. Heart—for heaven's sake, no! All this mushy and touchy-feely talk, I'd much rather remain where I am.

And could we now switch from my short legs to the length of the arms, please?

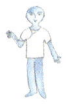

We could, but we won't. When you build a house you don't start with the roof. We will start to slowly and thoroughly establish the foundation.

You can just read the exercises. Though they're most effective if you take the time to do the whole course and participate in every step. Just like in *The Neverending Story*, you're a part of this book.

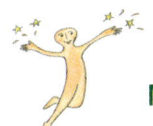
My body can talk

Wherever you are in this moment, stand up comfortably and tune in to yourself. Now sense:
your stance;
your breath;
the rhythm of your heart;
your aura;
your muscle tone;
and the rhythms in your body.

Allow yourself a few minutes for this exercise.

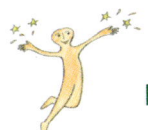
My body can say "yes" and "no"

Now, loudly say "yes", and feel what happens inside of you.
Then loudly say "no", and tune in again. When you say "no", does something change inside of you?
Repeat this exercise a few more times, alternating between "yes" and "no", until you're sure that what you feel is real and not an illusion.

You can also do this exercise sitting down if you feel embarrassed doing it while standing. However, in this case, I would suggest you repeat the exercise later standing up, since some things can only be sensed in this position.

Yes, you've perceived it right, there's a difference. Your body can indeed talk—and by the way, that's me who's talking—your inner wisdom.

I can:
make your muscles strong or weak;
make your breath light or heavy;
contract your energy field and expand it;
give you lightness and heaviness;
and much more.

And this is your lie detector, because every stress is palpable, it's a weight on one arm of your inner scale.

So I can say "yes" or "no," and I can warn you when you're going to do something that's not good for you; or I can empower you when you choose the right path.

That's enough for now.
I am like a lover—I want to be undressed slowly, very slowly. Take your time discovering me.

 And here is an inspiration for how you can effectively free yourself of deeply rooted behavioral patterns:

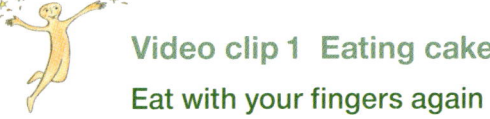

Video clip 1 Eating cake
Eat with your fingers again

When was the last time you ate using your fingers?

People in India always say that they can only really taste their food if they eat it with their fingers. Today you, too, will use your fingers, like a little child. If you prefer, you can go to a "dark restaurant" where people enjoy their meal in total darkness, where nobody can see it.

2.

LIFE ENERGY— THE MAGIC POWER

That was messy and yucky eating with my fingers. I didn't clean my fingernails before eating, and the food might be crawling with bacteria. So far, I don't have the runs, at least not yet.

For years, I've tried to control everything; I've tried to drive out the ill-behaved child, and then a book like this comes along. I consider this sabotage!

Hey, what are you babbling about, Mr. Mind? You want to sabotage? You did that far too long already, you party pooper. Whenever life gets ecstatic you come along with your reason, and the good energy is gone.

We'll talk later about who's actually doing the sabotaging here. But first, I want to know what this lie detector thing is all about.

You have no patience, do you? Are you afraid someone knows more than you? Or that someone could be able to find out if you speak the truth?

I prefer reason well done, so you may sizzle a bit longer in your own juice.

I thought about how I can make this book the ultimate healing experience for you.

To achieve this, let us use the power of manifestation. In my workshops, I've observed again and again how the wishes that the participants wrote down on the first day, manifested themselves at the end of the workshop. Create your own reality and simply write down your wishes in the following list:

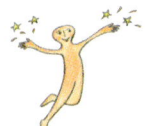

Make a wish

I let go of or want to change:
1. _____
2. _____
3. _____

I want to experience:
1. _____
2. _____
3. _____

What do you think, Doc? After all, aren't human beings just another kind of machine? And since there's no possibility of a perpetuum mobile, will you please explain to me what kind of energy it is that propels us?

Oh man, here we go, a real mechanic! Reminds me of what a woman in Mexico once said: "Our schools are from the 19th century, the teachers from the 20th century, and the students from the 21st century."

The outdated nonsense that our children still have to learn in school, for instance in physics and biology, is unbelievable. Only two years ago, a German physics teacher told a female student, who asked him a very simple question about quantum physics, that it would take him a few days before he could answer her question, since he himself had to look it up first.

Mr. Mind, here's your answer: The power is called life energy, and the conductors are, among others, the acupuncture meridians.

And for those of you who've already put mechanics in its place:

It's a magic power that gives us life.

It's also known as vitality, *prana*, *qi*, *orgone*, life force or simply life energy.

Its specialty: No technical instrument can measure it, no biophysicist can take out a patent on it, no schoolbook describes it, and yet, every human being knows about it.

Unfortunately, most people only learn to cherish it when they've lost it; when they feel run down, drained, tired, lacking strength, or are no longer able to perform, and then they blame it on getting older. Though in reality, age has nothing to do with it. There are children who have almost lost all their life energy, and 90-year-olds whose batteries are still full.

Without energy life becomes torture, and becomes simply about hanging on. If as a grown-up, you feel 20 years younger than your real age, you can be assured that you've got enough of this magic power. But if you feel as old in years as you are, it's time to charge the batteries again.

I've measured the life energy of thousands of patients, plus the energy levels of all acupuncture meridians. The energy patterns of the meridians corresponded exactly to the organic afflictions and basic problems of these patients. It's fascinating to see how the average value of the meridian measurements is equal to the amount of life energy. The following scale is the result of these measurements:

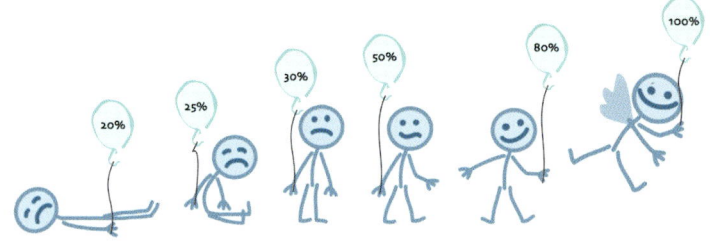

Life energy scale *(according to Uwe Albrecht)*

100%	Feels like flying or like falling in love
80%	Able to perform at full capacity, reaching your goals
70%	Normal productivity, but used to be better
50%	You're hanging in there, but it's not fun anymore.
40%	Productivity: 4 to 6 hours daily
30%	Exhausted after 2 hours of work, prone to tears
25%	Severe exhaustion, nothing matters anymore
20%	The battery is empty.

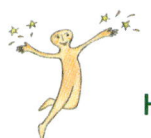

How high is your level of life energy?

What does your intuition tell you: How much life energy between 0 and 100 percent do you have right now? What's the first figure that comes to mind?

My life energy is: _____%

If you want to strengthen your life energy and enjoy its power, let your hands dance the *hand ballet*.

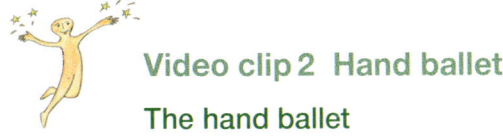

Video clip 2 Hand ballet
The hand ballet

Imagine you're deaf.

Though your hands can hear music and move in such a way that you feel the music with all your senses.

Now turn on the music.

Observe your hands and their ability to perceive the music, and their irrepressible zest to move accordingly.

After their first shy movements the hands get more and more courageous. They want to fill the room with their energy. The arms participate in the rapture and share in the dance. They dance in never before experienced swings, harmonies and twists. Sometimes slow, sometimes fast, and sometimes even stopping, like a maestro in front of his orchestra, with a quiet baton. Each hand finds its own mode of movement. Each finger discovers its uniqueness and acts it out.

The hands seize all reachable space; they can move easily above your head and behind your back. They're like dancers in a ballet. They tell their story using their own magic.

Once you've become enchanted by the beauty of your hands, close your eyes and let them dance again. Let them continue to revel in their newly found pleasure, lightness and freedom.

And then, if you feel like it, let your shoulders, your head, your pelvis, your belly and your energy field join the dance.

3.

THE ARM-LENGTH TEST—
TALK WITH YOUR SUBCONSCIOUS

Imagine that you can talk directly with your subconscious.
And that it responds to you.
That is the arm-length test.

I want. I want. I don't want to wait any longer.
You unwittingly subconscious darling, you just want to make me feel how little I have to say in these matters and how few shares I have.
I thought these kinds of stupid power games are my *line of work.*
Hey Missy, time to show me what you really know!

You really are so impatient, Mr. Mind! All in good time. We have to give the reader a chance to fling this book into the corner before we reveal the big secrets. Natural selection, if you will. Or do you believe the mystery schools will hand you the highest knowledge on a silver platter the moment you join them? First, the Doc will begin describing the lie detector so readers who are a slave to authority will keep silent.

I learned this test in 1996; but the osteopath Raphael van Assche discovered it many years before. He had pulled the arms of a patient who was lying down over her head to see if the muscle strands in both arms were of the same length. They were. But then the woman started to talk about her husband, and immediately the length of her arms differed. That's how it all began. Since then, thousands of therapists have worked with this test.

The test is a neurological reflex where the muscles on one side of the body tense up while being relaxed on the other side. Therefore, the length of the arms differs. This has to do with a particular neurotransmitter in the brain called substance P that controls the activity of our muscles. This substance is sent through our body at the unimaginable speed of 1,500 meters (about a mile) per second and results in either strong or weak muscles.

In my work as a medical doctor I use the arm-length test for everything: How is the condition of the inner organs? How high is the life energy? Which childhood trauma is not yet solved? Which medications help, which dental materials, etc. result in allergies? And does the person want to get healthy in the first place . . . ?

But I also test which sort of wine is good for me; which roads have police with speed radars on them (so I don't go faster than permitted); which t-shirt color is best for me, and so on. . . .

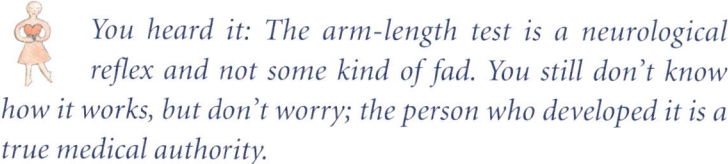

You heard it: The arm-length test is a neurological reflex and not some kind of fad. You still don't know how it works, but don't worry; the person who developed it is a true medical authority.

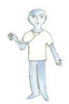 **Now you can learn the arm-length test step by step:**

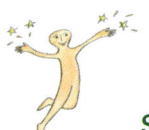
Step 1: Sensing colors

Imagine wearing clothing in different colors:

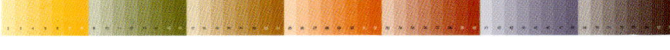

- Yellow
- Green
- Brown
- Orange
- Red
- Bue
- Purple
- White
- Black

Try to sense what each color does to you. Take a few minutes to find out.

Which color makes you feel good right now? Which color doesn't make you feel good?

And now, try this exercise again, with your eyes closed.

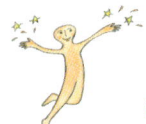

Step 2: I am a scale

Now stand up and imagine you're a scale.

Is the scale balanced or tilted?

If it's tilted, visualize now the different colors. Which color restores the balance? Once you have found the right color, put on a piece of clothing in that color or visualize doing it. It can be anything, even a shawl or a pair of socks.

If you can't find a color that balances your scale, take the one that was the most helpful and imagine different scents of essential oils.

Colors and scents together will most certainly balance your scale and make it straight.

Or you can follow your intuition and draw one to three healing cards from *The Complete Healing System*. Trust yourself, the card you draw is always the right one.

Continue reading *A Course in Healing* only after you have balanced your scale.

Congratulations, you have just treated yourself!

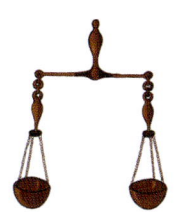 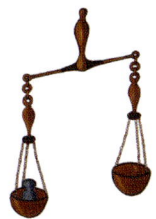 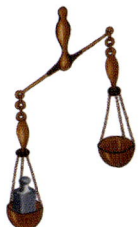

And since your scale is now straight, visualize putting a little weight in one of the pans, and notice how the scale moves. Next, put a heavier weight on, and then a very heavy one.

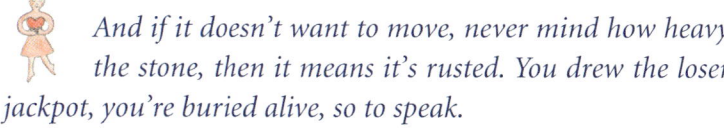
And if it doesn't want to move, never mind how heavy the stone, then it means it's rusted. You drew the loser jackpot, you're buried alive, so to speak.

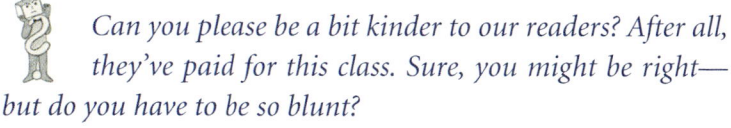
Can you please be a bit kinder to our readers? After all, they've paid for this class. Sure, you might be right— but do you have to be so blunt?

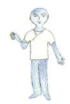 *Do you think life is going to say it to them in a kinder way when they're in a state of total rigidity, completely frozen in shock? Unsuccessful; not in contact with their own Self; suffering with cancer; or having accidents—is that kinder?*

After all, these are human beings, not sissies.

Actually the testing is very simple.

When we're in balance, the scale is straight.

If we're stressed the scale is tilted; like a scale with a weight in one of its pans.

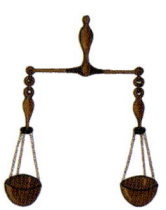
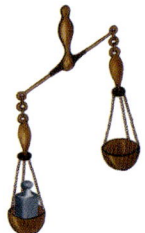

If we're in a state of rigidity, the scale doesn't move, regardless of whether it was straight or tilted when it entered that state. We're in a state of shock, as if we're frozen, lost in a trauma. And then not just the scale, but also time stands still for us.

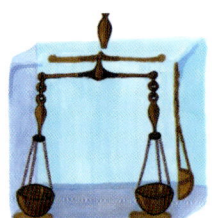
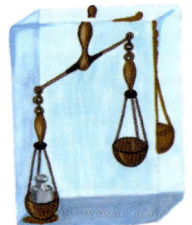

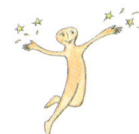

Video clip 3 The arm-lenght test
Step 3: The arm-length test

Let your arms hang loosely at your sides and relax your shoulders and arms.

Now let your arms meet gently in front of your body, right at your lower belly. Turn your thumbs outward in such a way that you can use your thumbnails as a measuring tool.

When you are in balance, your arms are equally long.

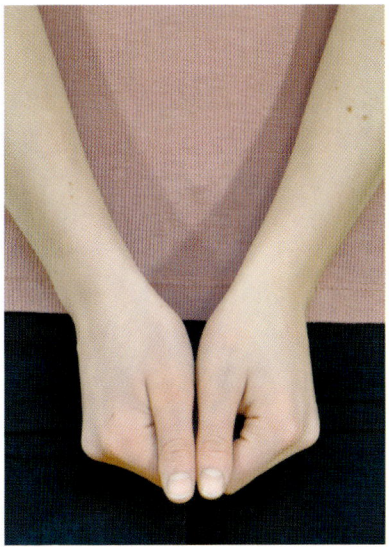

Take your arms back to the sides of your body.

Say "yes" once more and again bring your arms together in front of your body.

They will have the same length as before.

Now relax the arms one more time and let them hang loosely at your sides.

Say "no" and then bring the arms together in front of your body, like you did before.

This time the thumbs will not have the same length (unless you're in a state of rigidity, which I'll talk about later).

Your body says "no." It feels stress for having to say something negative.

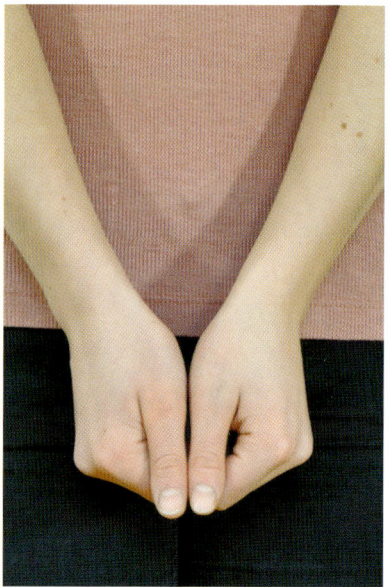 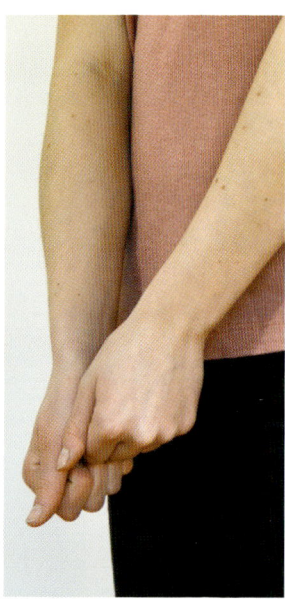

Now do the exercise again with your eyes closed. Frequently I close my eyes if I want to sense what's going on because we can often see better this way.

In the beginning, the difference in the lengths of our arms is often rather small, usually 0.5 to 1.5 inches. The more relaxed you are, the bigger the difference will be. Then even four inches are not uncommon. Just relax, and you'll get clear answers.

Once you reach a point where you don't mind what the answer of your thumbs is, you'll be a perfect tester.

Think about something positive: Your arms have the same length.
Think about something negative: Their length is different.

You have your stress and lie detector with you all the time.

Am I doing something wrong here? My scale says 'overload' though it's standing firmly on the ground. Could that be a kind of rigor mortis?

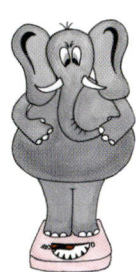

You're as good as dead. Or at least you're neither really alive nor able to test.

If your scale doesn't want to move, or if you don't get a "yes" or "no" response with your arms, or there's only a minimal difference, it means that you're in a state of rigidity.

The more flexible your regulation—your vibratory ability—the bigger the difference between the length of your arms will be when testing.

You can compare this with a windshield wiper: The more surface it cleans, the greater the clarity.

And here the emergency aid when blockages are present:

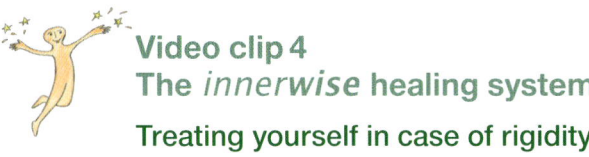

Video clip 4
The *innerwise* healing system
Treating yourself in case of rigidity

The arm-length test

Regular test

| Yes | No | Allergy/panic |

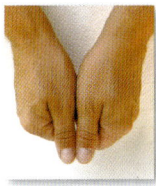 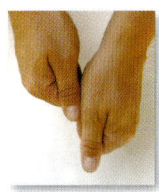 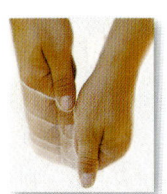

Initial stress ⇨ treat yourself

| Yes | No |

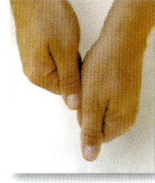 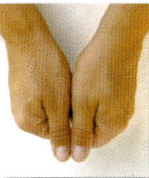

Blockage/rigidity ⇨ treat yourself

| Yes | No | | Yes | No |

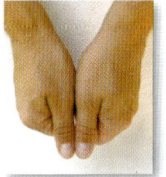 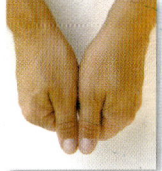 or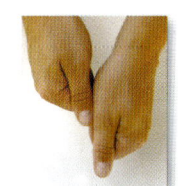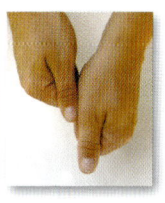

If you have access to *The Complete Healing System from innerwise*, intuitively draw one to five cards, which will open your ground regulation again. When testing with your arms now, you will again see differences. Don't worry; you will always draw the right cards. Now take the healing cards into your hands and let them do their work while you 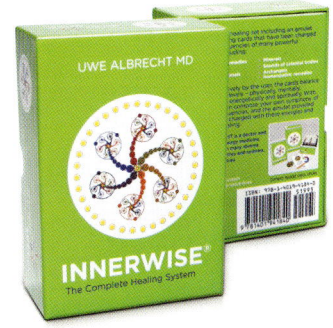 meditate with them for a few minutes. Then, copy them to the *innerwise* amulet of *The Complete Healing System* and wear it on a string above your heart.

If you don't have access to *The Complete Healing System*, you can treat yourself with the help of colors, herbs, scents, affirmations, prayers or music. When you choose the medium that is right for you, or just think about it, your blockages will disappear.

You always have the right remedies in your environment. Just trust.

When you're done, your arms will be of the same length if the answer is "yes," and of a different length if the answer is "no." Which shows that you have come back to life.

Self-treatment in case of rigidity and blockage

When you think of the proper remedy and visualize applying it, stress disappears and rigidity is dissolved.

Possible remedies are:

- Drinking water
- Changing the color of your clothes
- Imagining situations or colors
- Listening to music

- Speaking the truth
- Meditating
- Practicing yoga
- Painting or drawing
- Taking a shower
- Smelling flowers
- Drinking a cup of herbal tea
- Dancing
- Meditating with crystals
- Using Bach flower essences or homeopathy
- Going for a walk
- Treating yourself with *The Complete Healing System from innerwise*

Hey Doc, did you ever work with people who are in a coma, and where Mr. Mind, our logical mind, had no say anymore?

Yes, of course. It works beautifully. With the help of their arms one can talk with them and test what they need in order to wake up again.

I just read an article which said that it's possible to make brain reactions visible with the help of magnetic resonance imagining (MRI), and that doctors are glad to finally be able to communicate with their coma patients in this way.

But in reality, they were always able to do so. They just needed to take the patients' hands and ask them questions. Oh well, nowadays craftsmanship is rapidly losing its value.

Of course, coma patients could also respond (through their arms) that they would prefer not to wake up again, but rather, finally find peace.

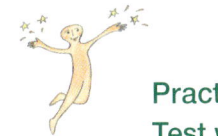

Practice, practice, practice: Test wherever you are

You now have the assignment to test with your arms as often as possible: while standing up, lying down, sitting, with your eyes open and with your eyes closed.

You can compare this with learning to play the piano, only this is much faster. The more you practice the arm-length test, the greater your trust in the results. Practice frequently with "yes" and "no" and test simple things, for example, test which colors you should wear that day.

Just say: "I'll wear something . . ." Then test, and your arms will say: "Yes, go for it." or "No, are you crazy?!?"

Please don't ask any questions about the future. It lies ahead of us and wants to be lived when the time comes. Since our present decisions can change the future any time, the arm-length test will not give us meaningful answers.

It also doesn't work to test lottery numbers.

If you test something, it's always a good idea to first ask the following questions:

"May I ask this question?"
"Will I get a meaningful answer?"

Some things are not for us to know—we have to experience them. With the help of these two questions you can prevent being misled by senseless answers.

The next chapter shows us the second part of the arm-length test: learning to see in a new way.

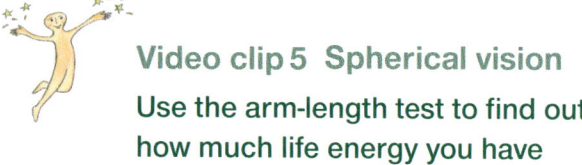

Video clip 5 Spherical vision

Use the arm-length test to find out how much life energy you have

Say: "I have 50 percent life energy." If your arms are equally long, your body says: "Yes, that's how much you have."

Then you say: "I have 60 percent life energy." If your arms are equally long again, this value is correct.

Now say 70 percent. Let's assume your arms now differ in length. In this case your body tells you: "No, you don't have 70 percent. You don't have that much energy left."

Now you can ask about 65 percent . . . continue asking and testing until you've determined the exact value.

If your arms already differed in length when you asked about 50 percent, you've got even less energy left. Then you ask about 40 percent, 30 percent . . . until again you find the exact value.

Now you know the amount of your present life energy.

My life energy is: _____%

I only have 30 percent. I feel bad, and according to your life energy chart I'm entitled to my depression.

You poor, poor victim!

What happened? Normally you can't wait to challenge everything. Maybe you should ask yourself where the remaining 70 percent has gone!

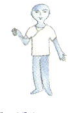 And now the definition of life energy for grown-ups; let's look at it from the perspective of self-responsibility.

100 percent of your energy is always available. Part of it gets used as life energy, which you have just tested, and part of it gets used as destructive energy. It's simple math:

100 − life energy = destructive energy.

Destructive energy is also active in you. It consists of all your compromises and lies; everything that you don't do because of fear. It's the energy with which you destroy yourself.

Combined, they always add up to 100 percent, and you decide how they're distributed between both sides.

> Calculation formular: 100 − life energy = destructive energy
>
> My destructive energy is: _____ %

 For some people, life is a chain of missed opportunities.

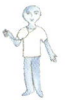 *Hey Doc, you forgot that I'm much more sensitive and can say way more with this arm-length test than just "yes" or "no."*

 Oh sorry, you're right.

You can say, it doesn't cause me any stress, or just a little, or a lot, or a huge amount of stress. And when you put your arms together several times, and they show an increasing difference, it means: "I am allergic." Or: "I am in a state of panic."

Yes or in balance

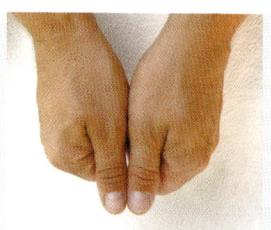

Very little stress,
very small "no"

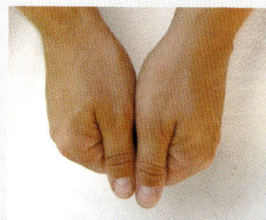

Medium stress,
Normal "no"

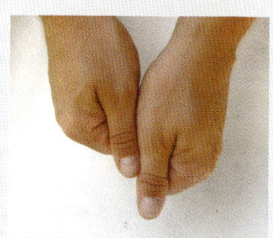

High stress,
big "no"

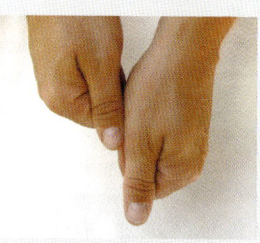

Very high stress,
huge "no"

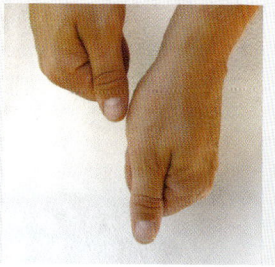

Allergy/panic

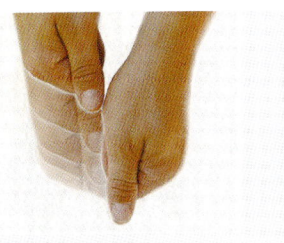

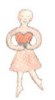
Very nice Doc. Now you only have to explain the difference between testing with statements or with questions. Then I'll be happy.

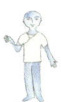
How can you assess the answers of the arms? It depends on what you're testing:

— In case you test statements like, "I do this . . .," equally long arms mean: "Balance. This is good for me."
Arms differing in length mean: "Stress. This is not good for me." And should the difference get bigger and bigger as you repeat the testing several times in a row: "It makes me wanna puke. This means allergy or panic."

Using statements, even as a beginner you can get reliable results.

— If you test with questions like: "Shall I do . . .?", "Will this . . . be bad for me?", assessing the response of your arms depends entirely on how you phrase your question. The arms can only say "yes" or "no."
Should it really be bad for you, your arms will be equally long and your body will say: "Yes, it will be bad for you, my dear." The allergy or panic response remains the same.

I recommend this version of testing with questions to those who are already confident in using the test, and who consider beforehand what a "yes" or "no" response means to them.

Assessment of the test response

Using statements

- Arms are equally long: Balance
  This is good for me.
- Arms differ in length: Stress.
  This is not good for me.
- The difference increases
  with repeated testing: Allergy or panic

Using questions

- Arms are equally long: Yes, this is right.
- Arms differ in length: No, this is wrong.
- The difference increases
  with repeated testing: Allergy or panic

4.

DO PEOPLE WHO ARE ILL WANT TO BE ILL

I feel it in my gut—today is my day! Today the minority shareholder is going to show the powerful a thing or two! To you, subconscious, you majority shareholder-sweetie: I want all people to be beautiful, rich, sexy, healthy and successful. Why does that seemingly not work? Who is sabotaging here?

Doc, I need your help for a moment.

With pleasure. Yes, there is a paradox here.

The patients come to me, they take half a day off from work, drive for hours, explain to me all the steps they've already taken, how many therapists they've worked with, and how much they've paid them in order to get well again. Then, I ask them to lie down and imagine being healthy, and promptly they're stressed. The arms differ in length and scream: "Oh no, not that!"

Then I ask them to visualize being ill, and the arms are equally long, which means: "Yes, I want that."

How will they ever get healthy if they can't even imagine it? Do they want it in the first place, or do they gain worthwhile benefits from being a victim?

Better keep it down, Doc. Or some clever tax officers will get the idea to equal "worthwhile" with monetary value and charge millions of Germans with tax fraud. They wouldn't even need to plant snitches in Swiss banks in order to steel the data. The hacking of health insurance funds' computers would be sufficient.

And how is the situation in regard to cancer patients, Doc?

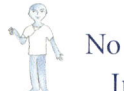 No difference.

In extreme cases when it comes to the statement, "I want to die," a cancer patient will say: "Yes."

"I want to live." "No."

If we're not able to stop this self-sabotage, the person will probably die soon, since a part of him or her wants to die.

And we always get the same results when using the arm-length test: People who are unsuccessful want to be unsuccessful. Unhappy people want to be unhappy; childless people want to be childless; and victims want to remain victims.

 So tell me, sweetie, who is really doing the sabotaging here?

IT'S ME. Though it's NOT sabotage.

Rather the old, unhealed hurts and pains stored inside of me. They want to be seen, cleared up, resolved and integrated. For me, it's only experiences that count.

And to get back to your cancer patient, Doc: What wants to die in this person is part of him or her, an unresolved trauma. Am I right, Doc?

Yes, you're right.

I almost always find this trauma (a separation, a loss, a deep hurt); it's something so painful that the person preferred to die instead of continuing to live.

And very often this kind of trauma happened a long time ago, perhaps even 10 to 20 years ago.

As a doctor, are you saying that people want to be ill, unsuccessful, unsexy and losers?

Yes, that's exactly what I'm saying; life unfailingly gives people what they wish for. This means they're fully responsible for their experiences. Their lives match their life plans and their ways of living.

So you honestly mean to say that each human being is responsible for everything that happens in his or her life? I always thought it's our parents' fault, the school's, the partner's, the preacher's, or the boss's. . . .
To think like that was so nice and easy; I could be angry at someone, work it out in therapy, and just be a victim.

Even Pippi Longstocking knew better:
"*Two times three makes four, deedle deedle dee and three makes niner, I can shape the world, howdle doodle doo I like it most!*" *(edited translation)*

[Translator's note: Since the English translation of the original varies greatly from the German version, a free translation was used to render the meaning that the author intended to convey with this quote.]

You don't really expect me to believe everything you just said?

No. I'll give you all the time you need to grow up.

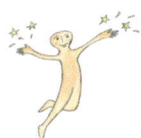
Now let's have a look at your basic programs:

31

The moment of truth

Stand up, relax your arms and shoulders, then say "yes," and bring your hands together in front of your body, right at the middle. Your arms should be equally long. Next say "no," and again bring them together in front of your body. Now the length of your arms should be different.

   For example, if your arms differed in length when you said "yes," or if there was no change at all when testing, please check the annex and treat yourself before you continue reading.

When everything works well, test the following questions and mark the answers immediately, without thinking about them:

The moment of truth
For testing and marking

I love myself:	Yes ○	No ○
I am honest:	Yes ○	No ○
I forgive:	Yes ○	No ○
I am healthy:	Yes ○	No ○
I am happy:	Yes ○	No ○
I am beautiful:	Yes ○	No ○

Okay, now I see what you mean.
But can I build on these answers; are they trustworthy? One can surely trick a little, right Doc?

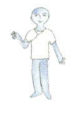 There is a way to get secure and reliable answers. By learning to see in a new way: by applying *spherical vision*.

You're accustomed to your own way of seeing

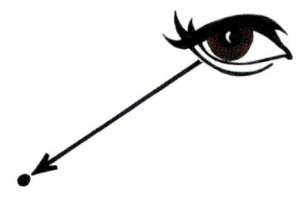

You look straight ahead. You look at a certain point. And you see from your own perspective based on your experience.

Spherical vision— the new type of vision

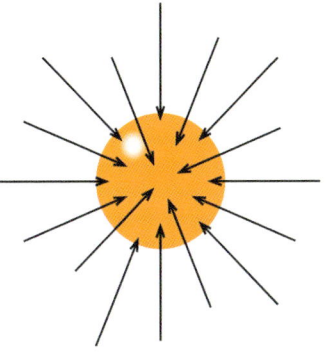

You look at something simultaneously from all directions. As though it's not you who sees, but *IT* that sees through your eyes.

Imagine you are the Earth and you could look at yourself from outer space.

In doing so, you notice that you're not a disc but a sphere, and that the Sun doesn't orbit around you.

St. Francis of Assisi described this kind of seeing with these words: "Lord, make me an instrument of your peace." *IT* sees through you, entirely free of judgment and prejudice.

 You're funny, Doc. After all, I consist almost entirely of judgment, prejudice and experience.

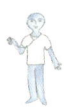 Then it's time you learn to see in a different way:

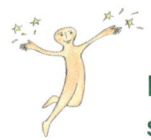

I can see something you don't see— spherical vision

Imagine you're standing at the edge of a sphere, and in the midst of it, there's a bouquet of flowers. You look at it from your direction. You can't see how the bouquet looks from behind, from above or from below.

Imagine you can see the bouquet from all section of the sphere. Now you can see everything.

How can you do this? It's very simple; don't look directly at the bouquet but at a point just before it, as if you want to see the aura, the energy field of the flowers.

This type of vision is a bit out of focus, and the eyes need to get adjust to it. And precisely this type of vision is the secret that you have to discover for yourself.

Now play a little more with both types of vision: the direct vision that you know, and the spherical vision. Repeat changing back and forth.

I know, the skeptic in each of us rebels in regard to this chapter. So my dear protagonists, one more time the most important question:

Why do people fall ill, Mr. Mind:

Because of viruses, bacteria and other beastly things, as determined by the genes; because of toxins in the environment; because this is what happens when we get older; because they've worked so much in their lives; because of the wicked cancer.

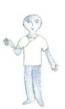 What do you say to that, Mrs. Heart?

 Wrong Mr. Mind. Most often people fall ill because they want to be ill.

 A tough statement, Mrs. Heart. Can you prove it?

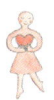 *Yes I can; blind, double-blind and triple-blind if you want, to satisfy all scientific criteria.*

Let's start with blind:

We take someone who is ill regardless of the illness, ask him to close his eyes, and use the arm-length test to check out the following statements:

"I want to be healthy."—This will generate stress; the answer is "no."

"I want to be ill."—This doesn't generate stress; the answer is "yes."

Now double-blind:

A therapist with his eyes closed tests the same questions using the patient's arms. The patient's eyes remain closed.
   The answers are the same.

And now a scientific novelty—triple-blind:

The patient is in a coma, his eyes are closed; the therapist's eyes are closed, too . . .
   The answers are still the same.

You can do the test with thousands of patients, and the results will always be the same.

– *Being ill: "Yes."*
– *Being healthy: "No."*

That raises a lot of questions, Mrs. Heart. Your argument suggests that a person's free will and intellect are meaningless.

5.

Journey through the Rhythms of the Body

The world is sound—Nada Brahma

Joachim-Ernst Behrend

This course follows a kind of logic that even I can understand. And I guess for now I have to accept the thing with the arm-length test, since I haven't yet discovered the trick hidden here. But I'll continue looking, and if I find it, I want to get more shares, at least 50 percent.

I would be happy if you finally could take additional shares, maybe 50 percent or even more. I won't stand in the way. Rid yourself of fear and negativity, and then you can have anything you want.

And now it's time Mr. Mind, to come out of your monkey cage since we have a surprise for you—we're going on a trip.

Yeah right, far away I hope. I would like to see something new for a change!

It's going to be a long trip into worlds unknown to you, and you'll work up a sweat, no doubt.

This exercise will help you to perceive yourself and other people, to sense where energy flows, where it's blocked, and how you and other people are doing in life.

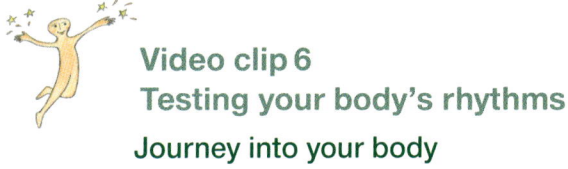

Video clip 6
Testing your body's rhythms
Journey into your body

Welcome to the world of your body.

Stand straight with your bare feet firmly on the ground. Relax your feet, your legs, your pelvis, your belly, your chest, your neck, your head, and visualize your favorite tree.

Feel its trunk, its branches, twigs, leaves and roots. Feel the sap in the tree rise, and imagine that you are this tree and the Sun is shining. You see clouds coming, rain trickling down on you, wind blowing at you.

Direct your attention back into your body.

Feel your feet and how they are standing on the ground. Notice if your weight rests on the ball of your foot, on the heel or in the middle. Sway a little to and fro and notice the changes. Compare your right and left foot; do they both carry the same weight, is the pressure the same on both feet?

Now direct your attention to your shoulders. Take a deep breath and focus your attention on the up and down movements of your shoulders: Are they the same on both shoulders? Continue breathing and compare the movements of both shoulders while taking deep breaths.

Feel your eyes. And stay completely focused on your eyes while visualizing the small muscles behind and around them. Now move your eyes a little and feel how these muscles are connected with other parts of your body.

Do you feel the movements of your eyes anywhere else in your body?

Feel the hair on your head, how it stands and falls together.

Imagine a down feather, and—beginning at the highest point of your head—use it to gently touch the centerline of your body: forehead, nose, chin, larynx, breastbone, navel, genitalia, anus, sacrum, and the spine back up again via the neck and on to the highest point of your head.

Now let the energy repeatedly circle around your body without the feather.

You realize that you are standing up, and you feel your thighs, and the power and tension in them. Feel your knees, your calves and your feet. Notice the pressure in your feet.

Is the pressure balanced, do both feet carry the same weight?

Sway again a little from the heels to the balls of the feet, and be aware of any changes in your body.

Take a deep breath through your nose. Was the breathing equally deep through both nostrils?

Continue breathing calmly and deeply and feel the air expanding through your lungs. Does it expand both lungs evenly?

Now take a very deep breath, and as you're breathing in and out, notice if the left and right sides of your chest rise and fall evenly.

Keep breathing calmly and feel if both shoulders rise and fall evenly while breathing in and out.

Breathe into your belly and pelvis. Feel how the breath expands and fills these parts of your body.

Breathe into your legs and down into the soles of your feet.

Now breathe into your head, your eyes and ears.

Breathe into your arms and hands.

Breathe in through your nose and breathe out through your genitalia: through the vagina or the penis.

Breathe in through your genitalia and out through your nose.

While you continue breathing in and out calmly, particularly notice the right and left sides of your body. Do both sides feel the same?

Really pay attention to how they feel.

Now hold your breath and focus on the right and left sides of your body.

Return to breathing calmly in and out through your nose, and direct your attention to the front and back of your body.

Now turn your entire awareness to the inside of your head.

All the bones of your skull are able to move a little, dancing with each other. You can sense the dance of each and every bone.

The energy flows down both sides of your head, and you feel your jaw joints, and the tension in them. Check if the tension is equal on both sides, then slowly open your mouth as wide as possible, and close it again. Notice if the movement goes straight down, or if the lower jaw slightly swerves to one side.

Feel all your teeth and notice how each tooth is connected to a particular part of your body. Start with your upper jaw and feel each tooth separately. Take your time so you can perceive the energetic connections.

Now turn your focus to the uppermost bone of your spine, feel how your skull rests on it. Consciously move down your vertebrae one by one and sense the mobility in each of them.

When you get to your tailbone, let it dance, very gently. Does it want to move in all directions?

Push your pelvis slightly forward, then backward, and feel the changes in your whole body.

Now you can sway again on your feet, from the heels to the tips of your toes, and notice the changes in your body.

With your whole body sway to the right and left and notice how it feels.

Can you hear your heart? Feel it, feel its rhythm.

Feel the rhythm of your lungs, your breath.

Feel the rhythm of your skull.

Feel the rhythm of your liver, feel how it breathes.

Now feel your kidneys, feel how they breathe.

Now you are ready to feel yourself in a new and profound way.

Notice the symphony of the different rhythms of all your inner organs, your entire body.

Take deep breaths in and out every part of your body; from the tip of your hair, to the soles of your feet.

Take your time to nourish all areas of your body with the most loving breath you've ever caressed them with.

6.
Do we get sick from viruses or bacteria?

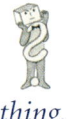 *Where is my breathing mask? Help, the viruses are coming! Stay away from me; I don't want to catch anything.*

As I've explained to you before, there are other reasons why a person falls ill. Are you suffering from your anxiety neurosis again, Mr. Mind?

What do you mean, "anxiety neurosis"? Every child knows—and every medical book confirms it—that one gets sick from viruses, bad bacteria and fungi.

 Oh, those poor bad, bad things!
Who do you think makes your beer, your bread, your wine, and who produces vitamins in your intestines? Who turns a hamburger into something digestible? All those bad things, that's who.

What about the streptococci, which are responsible for tonsillitis and which I kill off with antibiotics?

To get rid of these bacteria you have to practically incinerate yourself. Then you'll get rid of them and all your problems, for good.
Sorry, but I have to challenge your ego again today, Mr. Mind.

There are ten times as many germs in the intestines as cells in your body. If we established democracy now, even the best lobbying couldn't help you, Mr. Mind.

As long as you live, there'll be streptococci in your mouth and yeast fungi in your intestines. . . .

 Then what makes me sick, smarty pants?!?

All right you squabblers; let me explain!

About 45 years ago, there lived some very wise men in Vienna, Austria, who revolutionized modern medicine, but today they're almost forgotten. They realized how illness originates, and how healing can occur. All of this was forgotten as soon as the miracle weapons of medicine entered the stage: antibiotics and cortisone.

Reflecting and deliberating were not called for anymore, and neither was understanding—instead, the order of the day was: Here's a pill, have a nice day!

Those wise men were—among others—Mr. Pischinger and Mr. Perger, both professors at universities in Vienna. They showed that health is based on free ground regulation, or the role connective tissue plays and the fact that illness begins with blockages and the build-up of waste products in connective tissues.

A healthy person is a person in harmony, as harmonious as a beautiful sinus curve. Then a shock, trauma or injury occurs, and the beautiful sinus curve changes into a straight line.

Like in the movies when a beautiful heroine dies in the emergency room, and instead of the sine wave the monitor shows nothing but a flat line.

In this state you're practically dead—trapped in you own body. Your access to yourself is lost. You see the world through a layer of fog, and time becomes unreal. "What, summer is almost over?!?" would be a typical perception of time in this condition.

Since this state of being is unbearable, the body tries to break through the rigidity: fever, the sniffles, diarrhea, accidents ... the body stops at almost nothing to try and get moving again. The goal is to create chaos at all costs to help you awaken from the rigidity. That is the reason why little children suddenly develop a fever at night, only to be well again in the morning. The fever helps the child to break through a state of rigidity.

In this way the body attempts to heal itself. Sometimes it prefers to overshoot the goal a bit instead of having to live with the rigidity; rigidity is not livable.

Are you saying that all those beastly little things like viruses, bacteria, fungi and whatever they're called, help the body to get out of its state of rigidity?

Yes, you got it right. These "beasty little things" help the body by creating a snotty nose, abundant diarrhea and a hot fever. Or they open the skin if too much filth has accumulated underneath. . . .

Do people in a state of rigidity always experience complete failure? There are many people who are blocked in one way or the other, but still move around quite lively, aren't there?

Think of a windshield wiper—if it cleans the window perfectly, we can relax and sit comfortably, see everything in front of us and enjoy driving.

Now imagine that the windshield wiper cleans only half of the window. That's the end of fun driving. True, you can still fly across the Interstate at 90 miles an hour, but the danger to bump into something to your left or right is greater. And when the windshield wiper only cleans a little space in the middle of the windshield you'll anxiously lean forward to stare through the peephole.

When it stops working altogether you can lean back again comfortably, relax and say good-bye, since the only question is which tree will make itself available for your departure and deliverance.

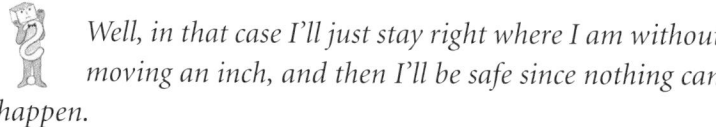
Well, in that case I'll just stay right where I am without moving an inch, and then I'll be safe since nothing can happen.

Great idea, most people do exactly that: standstill, gridlock, don't move, breathe sparsely and hope for better times. But they don't understand what's happening to them. They wonder why nothing seems to work in their lives anymore. No more energy. No more zest for life. They stumble through life with blinders.

One night last winter, when I had to drive home from a workshop, it was so cold that the windshield washer fluid was frozen despite antifreeze. I was on the freeway with smeared windows, snowdrift and useless windshield wipers at below 0 degrees Fahrenheit. It was an absolute worst-case scenario. When I got home I was totally exhausted and had barely survived the trip. The only reason I made it home safely was the fact that I was able to maintain my inner harmony.

Besides, before any accident the people in question find themselves in a state of rigidity regarding their ground regulation.

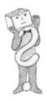
Why?

Because our response time multiplies, our guardian angels don't work properly, and we lose access to our inner voice.

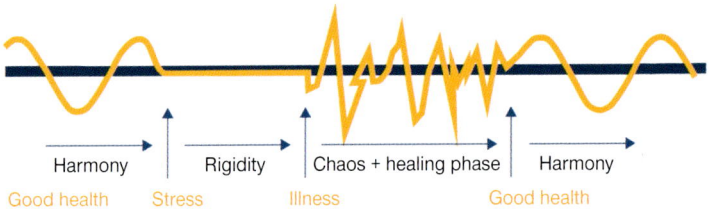

Harmony	Rigidity	Chaos + healing phase	Harmony
Good health	Stress	Illness	Good health

Let's summarize one more time:

When we're healthy, we're in harmony like a beautiful sinus curve.

But when stress happens, or shock, we become rigid, and partly or totally paralyzed. Our sinus curve stretches into a flat line.

Now the body attempts a healing reaction: sniffles, cough, diarrhea, fever and sometimes even an accident. It doesn't fuss with *what* and *where*—the main thing is to create chaos in order to break through the blockage. And now the hour has come for the "beastly little things," since they help the body reach its goal. This is the moment where according to conventional medicine illness begins, whereas in reality they've already missed the first and second act of the drama.

When the chaos has tidied up enough and everything goes well, health and harmony are restored.

But it's possible that things don't go so well, meaning the person doesn't get back into harmony, but stays in chaos. Then we have a chronic illness, which indicates that the original rigidity is not yet dissolved.

When we succeed to perceive, test and treat the rigidity, the flat line, and in that way resolve it, we can spare ourselves the chaos of the healing reaction. We abbreviate and jump directly to *Go!*

Here is another example from my experience:

A woman comes into my practice, 52 years old, and tells me she would finally love to learn a profession.

Among other questions I ask her if she knows how to play an instrument. She says: "Yes, the guitar." Then I ask her when the last time she played it was. "When I was seventeen," she says.

One more time, just to make sure you caught that: *She says she plays the guitar, and the last time she played was 35 years ago.*

Where have all those years disappeared to; what did she do with them?

Hustling to make a living, a few occasional jobs, and that's it—the balance sheet of 35 years of human life.

To be honest, in many people's lives the balance sheet looks pretty similar: **I've survived.**

Because of a trauma at the age of 17 this woman had fallen into a state of total rigidity and didn't wake up for 35 years.

Thankfully, most cases don't develop into situations as extreme as this one.

Though at least 30 percent of all human beings are in a state of rigidity; sometimes for hours, sometimes for days, and sometimes for even longer.

> **Therefore ground rule no. 1:** Never remain in a state of rigidity. Take a break and treat yourself.
> With the arm-length test, *The Complete Healing System* from *innerwise* with its test cards and the healing cards it's really easy to do.

7.

Let's try saying "thank you!"

If we want to heal all wounds, in many cases we can try a therapeutical approach. At the end of the journey lies a very simple solution—feeling gratitude for the experiences. This is healing in itself.

　Today we will practice saying "thank you."

　Thank you. Thank you. Thank you. What can be so difficult here that we have to practice it?
Thank you, God, for this glorious day. Thank you for my beautiful body. Thank you for the flowers.
It starts to get boring.

　All right then, I'll challenge you a little more:
Say "thank you" and feel it.
Imagine saying "thank you" while you're looking into someone's eyes; and imagine saying "thank you" while you're looking into someone's heart.

　That's something I can't do on my own. You are in charge of feelings, so you better help me with this!

　Okay, I will help you. Imagine someone who, a long time ago, has hurt you a little!

Imagine looking into that person's eyes while saying "thank you," and imagine looking into his or her heart and saying "thank you."

It's high time you stop torturing the readers and me. Why this nonsense? What am I saying "thank you" for? I'm not thankful that someone hurt me!

Imagine someone in your life who has hurt you a little more! Imagine saying "thank you" while looking into the eyes of that person, and imagine saying "thank you" and looking into the heart of that person.

You just go on without listening to me. . . .

Imagine the person in your life who has hurt you more than anybody else ever! Imagine saying "thank you" while looking into the eyes of that person, and imagine saying "thank you" and looking into that person's heart.

You're a sadist.

Maybe you'll fly into a rage.
  But do you really believe that I want you to be thankful for the pain? By now you should know me a little better. What happened to your trust?
  I haven't told you yet what you should be thankful for.
  I only ask you to be thankful because every time you got hurt you were allowed to learn something.

I've never met a patient in my practice who has never been hurt in his or her life.

Everyone, at one point or another, has felt one or more of the following: not being a wanted child, parents' fears that get transferred to their children, sadistic teachers, lost lovers, the deaths of loved ones, self-mutilation because of unfulfilled expectations and much more....

No matter the injury or hurt we have experienced, there are always two steps necessary to heal them:

1. Gratitude for the experience, however painful it was.
2. Retrieving the part/s of us, of our soul, which we've lost due to the hurt. In a few moments I'll show you how to do that.

I also work with the *Weißer Ring*, an organization that helps victims of violence. I've meet with people who have suffered serious traumas. They've been brutally battered, abused or blackmailed. When we meet for the first time, the traumatic experience usually happened about three weeks prior. All of these people are trapped in a state of total rigidity, as I described in the previous chapter. Time has stopped for them the moment they got hurt or traumatized.

For these people, too, the only possibility for healing is the two previously mentioned methods: gratitude for the experience, and the retrieval of the lost soul fragments.

Then miracles can happen.

Once I had a female patient whose ex-partner had tried to strangle and kill her ten days before. He had broken into her house at night, and she barely survived the attack. After one hour of therapy work she was able to imagine looking him into the eyes again and, while remaining strong, thanking him for all her experiences, to sense him clearly, and to understand which old traumas had broken him. She could even imagine sleeping alone again in her house, with the windows open and without fear. When she first came to me, she trembled with fear; when she left, she was calm and relaxed.

This is very thrilling work—even authors and film directors have sat in on treatments to draw inspiration from them.

A few more minutes until we start working on gratitude. First, I want to show you some tools that will help you to heal yourself, without the drama and return of the pain.
All of the images in the following section "The river of life" came to life during treatments.
Nothing is as thrilling as life itself!

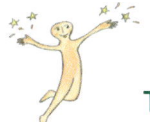

The river of life

Retreat to a quiet place and find your inner peace. Sit or lie down comfortably.
Close your eyes and take a few deep breaths.

Now visualize before your inner eye the color blue. Notice how this blue is starting to move, to form waves, to become water and to flow along like a river.
Look into the river and now recognize your own reflection in it.
You see a boat in the river. It is your boat.
You are in your boat and right in the center of this river.

Take a look around you—you see the shore, the meadows and the trees—and notice the river and see how the leaves are floating on the surface of the water.

Now notice the direction in which your boat is going. Are you going to the source or to the mouth of the river? If you are going to the mouth, think about why your boat is heading in this direction.

Think back to times in your life when you moved toward the source.

If you are going to the source, think about why your boat is heading in this direction.

Notice how much you have to struggle against the current in order to get closer to your destination.

Look around you and see all the other boats going in the opposite direction.

Haven't you asked yourself all along why your life consists of so much struggle and loneliness?

You now have the opportunity to learn how to trust. Change the direction, allow yourself to drift along—to be in the flow.

Now come back into the present moment and see what is inside your boat. Is there anybody else coming along for the ride?

If so—it may be an animal, a partner, friends or your children—look the animal or the person into the eyes and ask them: "Why are you in my boat?", "Why are you not sitting in your own boat?", "Who invited you?", "Do I need you in my boat?"

Notice if you are sitting in the front or in the back of your boat. Are you at the helm, or did you surrender control to someone else who is now steering your boat?

Imagine how it feels to be alone again in your boat; to navigate alone, perfectly at peace with yourself.

Now the time has come for the other individuals or animals to leave your boat and enter their own that is gliding along beside yours. Imagine how they are leaving the boat. And if there is something that is holding them back, imagine a color that envelops them so that they can leave.

Now you are again alone in your boat.

Your partner, your friends, your children, your pets—whoever is in your heart is right beside you traveling in their own boat.

And there are passages in the river where your boats are drifting apart a little, and other passages where you are coming closer together again. There are no anchors or ropes between you and the others. You trust that it is right exactly as it is in any given moment.

You are watching all the other boats on the river and notice how two boats that were close together separate, and how at a fork in the river each boat is going its own way.

This fills your heart with great joy and gratitude—you see that two human beings spent a part of their lives together, and have taught each other what they had agreed to teach each other before they stepped into their boats. Now they separate and set each other free, so they both can keep growing and have the opportunity to fulfill other contracts that they agreed upon.

Suddenly you hear it.

There it is, this rushing noise somewhere ahead of you. And it is getting louder. Now you know what it is—a waterfall. You look around, there is no chance you can pass it;

you are drifting closer and closer. Are you afraid? If so, which star or planet is coming to mind right now? Ask it to give you strength and courage and trust so you can drive directly into the waterfall. Slowly count to three and feel how your boat flies and lands softly on the other side of the waterfall. You are amazed to see that your fear was unnecessary, and you remember situations in your life where the fear was stronger than your courage, and how this deprived you of wonderful experiences.

Now you know that with the help of stars and planets you can conquer any waterfall.

The river is getting very still, and twilight is approaching. You hear the bird's lovely evening songs; in a bay candles are floating on the water, and you feel a deep desire for closeness, an embrace and a union with another human being. If something is holding you back now and doesn't allow for this deep desire, imagine a crystal, its color, its form; become one with the crystal and feel how a deep sense of peace is arising in you. And now feel the desire for melting with another person in you.

Your boats are blending and become one, and you both begin to merge into one another. With your eyes, your touch, your kiss you are diving deeply into each other and you feel how you become one joint breath. The most wonderful energy is arising in both of you, your breath becomes ever more intense, and you are filled with a feeling of infinite bliss and completeness, time- and spacelessness.

Dusk is falling already, and time has come to move on. Look at your boat—it is changing into a kayak. And you see a sign hanging above the water:

"Caution, whitewater! Only one boat at a time."

Before you have time to think the current is pulling your boat into rough waters. The water is churning, gushing over boulders, and you are getting caught in wild swirls.

You are doing well; you are mastering the challenges. But suddenly the water capsizes your boat. You are hanging on to your kayak with your head under water. The water has overpowered you. You feel the air getting less and less. It may last another 30 seconds, not more. You have to make a decision. You can leave the boat, or try to turn it around to get above water.

An inner voice tells you: Try it, you can do it, turn yourself around. You do try it, but to no avail. Time is running out. Living or dying—again the choice is yours: to leave the boat, or to summon every ounce of your strength and try again. Yes, you did it! Your head is above water again. You feel the fresh air, and how it fills your lungs. You are alive!

The water quiets down again, and you see a wall in front of you. All the water shoots through a hole in this wall. What is behind it? An abyss? The end? Paradise? You don't know, and you can't find out, unless you trust and flow with the water through this hole.

You could also wait at the shore, stare at the hole every day of your life and see how all the other boats drive through it. Years of your life, wasted because of fear. Didn't you do that too many times already? And in the end it will be the same as with the waterfall—very easy.

This time you trust and drive through.

And then . . . you find yourself on the most beautiful, blue, quiet lake. The Sun is shining, fish are playing in the water, and you are looking back at the hole. It is not there anymore, now there is only a window. And above the window are written the words "window of gratitude." You can only see those experiences in your past for which you are grateful.

You are standing in front of this window looking through it. What do you see? And what don't you see?

It's not easy to say "thank you" for hurts, pain, fear, loneliness or losses.

All of a sudden you notice radiant light coming toward you. You sense it inside yourself and you hear a voice—a clear, innocent voice that tells you: *It's easy; you have planned your life exactly as it is, with all the experiences you've had. And these experiences have enriched your soul. They've made you what you are today: wonderful, lovable and a little wiser.*

Think about your entire life and say: "Thank you for giving me the opportunity to have all of those experiences." Repeat it again and again, until you can see your whole life in your window of gratitude.

You don't know how much time you've spent in front of this window; it seems like an eternity even though it was only a few moments. And you made it! Your heart feels light and free, you are filled with a power you thought you had lost forever. Yes, you are born again, and you have become wiser. And with this inner richness you can now help others who still see themselves as victims in their lives.

Again, you find yourself sitting in your boat. The current of the lake propels you further on. You are looking ahead but you can't see very far because there is a fog so dense that you can't even begin to guess what awaits you ahead.

By now you have already embarked on the unknown so often that this time you feel a joyful expectation, a tingling, similar to the delicious feeling you had as a child just before Christmas. Which gifts are waiting for you now?

You are diving into the fog, gliding along. Suddenly you see a wild swirl of water in front of you. You have no choice—the entire lake gets pulled inside into it.

It's a hole—a black, infinitely deep and quiet hole.

You are jumping into nothingness.

And it is the most magnificent thing you have ever experienced in your life. You are everything, and nothing, human being and God, you are flying like you always have been able to in your dreams. You are one with everything, limitless, infinite. You experience a profound transformation. You become enlightened and find yourself again at the source of the river. The river of love, and your boat of life is ready for a new journey.

But first you rest a while and think about your last journey on the river. Just now you remember how you always wanted to go *against* the current; you think of all the sweating and puffing, and you have to laugh at yourself. You remember all the boats you saw, the boats with your ex-partners, your partner and children sitting there beside you. There was one boat where the partner was tied up with chains so he would not disembark. Now you can laugh heartily about your fear at the waterfall. And you still feel the shared breath of love inside of you. How blessed human beings are to have a body to experience all this.

The whitewater with the hole at the end, the beautiful lake lost in a fog, and this fantastic maelstrom of water that you jumped in head first—all of that you remember with gratitude.

This journey was, once again, a really good one.

Now you decide to rest a little and to make sound plans for your next journey on the river, to find friends who will participate so that at the end of your new journey, you can laugh again joyfully at yourself.

And the time will come when you will embark on a new boat again. . . .

8.

I AM YOUR SYMPTOM

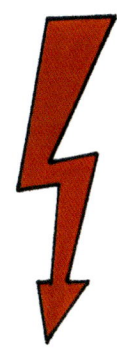

*They call me **symptom**. I have many names: knee pain, pimples, stomachaches, rheumatism, asthma, snot, depression, migraine, hemorrhoids, and the list goes on and on.*

I have volunteered for the worst possible job: being the bearer of unwelcome tidings.

Nobody understands me. They all think that I want to annoy them, slow them down, hurt them or restrict them. This is complete nonsense.

I simply try to speak with them in a language they understand. Would you go negotiate with the barbarians at the gates with a flower in your hand and a "Peace" t-shirt on your back?

However, most people don't understand me. They hit me with a sledgehammer—the largest they can find. "Shut up!" they say, and "Will you be quiet!" This is what I have to hear time and again. Then they put me on drugs: sleeping pills or antidepressants. They try and tape my mouth shut. Some people get really creative in their responses.

Meanwhile, all I want is what's best for them.

Imagine that I am the alarm siren on the Titanic warning about an iceberg. . . and everybody who hears me just complains that I'm keeping them up.

A pipe is broken in a classroom, and the water level is rising, but the teacher doesn't notice. A child gets up and screams for help. So what does the teacher do: He takes a gun and shoots the child because he or she has disturbed the lesson, and the teacher *can't take the screaming. Now none of the other children dares to say anything and everyone drowns.*

Does that make it any clearer?

I'm the child who dared to stand up and scream.

You think I am "THE ILLNESS." Nonsense. Do you know what THE ILLNESS really is? It's you and your way of life.

This must come as a shock, I know. It's OK if you're feeling a bit upset right now. I can handle your process quite well. In fact, it's part of my job. The good news is that it's up to you to no longer need me.

When I enter your life, what you should really do is put your angry reaction on hold and ask yourself: "What is this telling me? Why am I getting this now? What do I have to change so that I no longer need it?"

If you leave the work only to your mind, the response won't get you any further than it has in years past. However, if you ask your subconscious, your heart, and also use the arm-length test, you will get very clear answers that truly help you move forward.

And if you take care to stay in balance you can shorten many of my visits or do without them.

Put me out of a job! Or do you still think I really like this kind of work?

In order for you to understand my messages better, here is a little dictionary that helps you translate them:

••• (If you want to know more about the translations of "symptom messages," I suggest the book *Metamedizin* [or *Métamédecine* or *La Metamedicina* or *Metamedicina*] by Claudia Rainville. Unfortunately, this book was not available in English at the time of publication, but if you can read in German, French, Spanish, or Italian this book can be very helpful to you. Also, if you can only read in English there is another book with similar information, written by Louise Hay, called "Heal Your Body.") •••

Symptom	Meaning/message
Gas:	Too much food or food intolerance.
Bellyache:	Something I haven't digested; something I've swallowed; rage. (The Chinese diagnose bellyache as: The overpowering liver—rage—strangles the center.)
Pimples:	Emergency cleansing to get rid of toxins.
Sniffles:	I'm sick and tired of something. Enough already!
Heavy feet:	Standing still. Having lost mobility.
Backache in the morning:	I'm sleeping in a bad place.
Sneezing:	Energetic cleansing.
Headache:	Being under pressure.
Knee pain:	Am I going in the right direction?
Cardiac arrhythmias:	Having lost one's rhythm.
Inflammation of the middle ear:	Milk protein intolerance
Cancer:	A part of me wants to die.
Depression:	My life is full of energy-devouring compromises
Heart pain:	Love has died long ago; or I allow someone to feed him- or herself on my heart energy.

Our symptoms are not always messages for *us*. Approximately 30 percent of all illnesses or disorders that we carry are for other people. "A sorrow shared is a sorrow halved." Says the deeply internalized, stupid slogan of our ancestors.

Because of misinterpreted love, "helper syndrome" or through manipulation we adopt other people's issues as our own. Then, the message of the symptom advises us to finally cherish ourselves enough to know that our own well-being is more important than the well-being of other people. With healing work we release the load—that is, the energetic charges—that we carry for others, and trust them again to solve their problems themselves. Only in this way can people change something in their lives and grow.

Once a female patient came to me suffering from a lack of energy (compromises lived in life), high blood pressure (being under pressure). Testing revealed that these were not her issues but someone else's. Then she talked about a friend who has problems with her mother, her siblings, her partner and her job. "I am sorry for her and I would do anything to help her feel better," my patient added.

I translated her words for her: "I cause myself harm, and am even willing to fall ill or die from this illness, if it means that this will make her feel better."

Her sacrifice is not of any help to her friend; only she herself, who has the problem, can change her life to feel better again. However, if her friends take the pressure away from her, and she feels better because of that, the necessity to clean up her life is no longer there.

We all need a certain amount of pressure or suffering to help us let go of supposed security and sort out our lives.

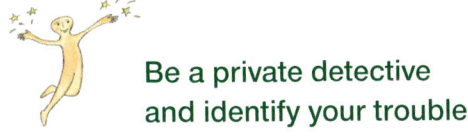

Be a private detective and identify your troubles

Use the following list to write down your symptoms, pains and illnesses.

1. Now test the following for each point on your list: "Is it my issue?"

   Answer "No":
   "Do I carry the issue for someone else?"
   "For whom?"
   "Does it help the other person if I carry it?"
   "Am I allowed to let it go, so the other person clears it up on his or her own?"

   Answer "Yes":
2. When did the issue behind the symptom begin?
   Test in which year, month . . . the reason first appeared.
   If you know the time of its first appearance, you probably can easily connect it with a specific experience.

3. Test which issue is the cause of the symptom.
   Just test different questions: Is my symptom connected to . . . ?
   If the body says "yes," i.e., your arms are equally long, then you've found the connection, or part of it.

4. Can I let go of the symptom—my aid worker? Have I already understood the message?

If the answer is "no," and the length of your arms differs, ask yourself:
"How much longer do I need the symptom?"

If the answer is "yes":
Test what helps you and treat yourself with colors, herbs, oils, teas, music, *The Complete Healing System* from *innerwise*, homeopathy, etc.

Symptoms, irritations, illnesses	It's my issue Yes/No	I carry the issue for . . .	The issue started (day/month/year)	It's related to . . .	I am ready to let it go Yes/No	Remedy

Don't be disappointed if testing was a bit difficult right now. It's like learning to play the piano; eventually it becomes natural. And *eventually* will be very soon, in the next few days, if you practice regularly and don't forget to apply spherical vision.

 Let me tell you a little story about Hannes:

After his parents' separation, Hannes and his siblings spent two weeks with their mother and two weeks with their father each month. Both parents lived in the same vicinity so this arrangement didn't cause any problems. In fact, it's a wonderful solution, even if the old-fashioned ladies at the youth welfare offices throw their hands up in horror. (It's time to transfer these ladies to a nursing home.)

With this kind of equally shared care for their children, Hannes' mother and father were able to impart their values, raise their children and share their lives with them.

Last winter, the children went on a ski holiday with their mother. Hannes was 15 years old, and when they got back home he complained about knee pain and numbness in his feet.

It all began after a confrontation with his mother, which was so unbearable for the boy that he disappeared for a few days. He felt misunderstood, controlled, and he couldn't feel her trust.

Then Hannes wrote a letter to his mother where he emptied his heart and bared his soul; he was finally able to express his feelings.

The moment the letter disappeared into his mother's mailbox, the pain in his knees was gone, and he could feel his feet again.

9.

innerwise®:
THE COMPLETE HEALING SYSTEM
SELF-TREATMENT FOR EVERYONE

You probably own a computer, use the Internet, can access information and know how to copy data and send pictures all over the world.

Do you ever ask yourself how all of this works? If you are like the majority of us, you probably don't.

Now imagine that all of this can work without hardware, computers, servers, cables and programs.

You can connect with a network, download information and exchange energies, see images from far away regions, copy data, and let frequencies do their work inside your body.

Now you've arrived at *innerwise*, an intelligent energy system. It sounds like a pie in the sky, but it's actually already available now.

Do you have any questions about how it works? The only thing missing, when compared with the computer version, is the comprehensible hardware.

Instead, there is the human being with his limitless capabilities of which until now we have only used a fraction.

The healing cards, of which 309 are included in *The Complete Healing System* from *innerwise*, enable us to work with 309 different information patterns.

The Complete Healing System contains the patterns and energies of homeopathic remedies, Bach flower essences, Schuessler tissue salts, animals, herbs and many more. In technical terms, all of these energies are complex information patterns that are characteristic for each of these remedies. Access to these patterns is made possible through the geometric structures and numbers on the healing cards, like a destination address in a database. The cards are the gateway to the frequencies so to speak.

I have established the actual database with more than 4,000 *innerwise* frequencies in energy field structures. I don't expect you to understand all of this at once. Even for me it's often a journey into unknown worlds. It's part of my life purpose to manifest *innerwise* in the world and make it accessible to many people.

I grew up an atheist. However, thanks to the work with *innerwise*, I was allowed to discover the existence of a principle of Creation, and the fact that this principle is capable of manifesting itself through us to guide our lives. As the physicist Werner Heisenberg once said: "The first gulp from the glass of natural sciences will turn you into an atheist, but at the bottom of the glass God is waiting for you."

Of course, one may exclaim now, "But that's not really possible. How did you get your knowledge?"

Not long ago, human beings believed that the Earth was a disc. Even if *innerwise* seems to be a bit ahead of its time, it doesn't mean that it doesn't work.

For me, there's only one criterion that matters: Does it work?

And the answer is yes, it does (even if we don't yet completely understand *how*). The system works for individuals as well as with animals, companies or organizations, and projects that don't ask comprehension questions. Do you really understand how electricity moves through a cable made of dense matter?

I don't. No explanatory model has truly convinced me thus far. Nevertheless, we use electricity.

Human beings sense the energies of the healing cards and can even describe them; they immediately feel their effectiveness as a remedy. Illnesses and problems disappear with their support. We can test them using the arm-length test. For me, that's all the proof I need.

In the last years, I've raised the energy of the entire *innerwise* system. Our consciousness was ready to work with stronger energies. Many *innerwise* mentors in different countries sensed that change without knowing that I'd done so. They felt the difference. When I made some energetic changes in Berlin, in the very same moment the *innerwise* system in Vancouver, Mexico City, Vienna, Dresden and The Hague also changed.

Onetime we energetically copied regular blood pressure pills. When the copies were given to patients they produced the same effect as the real pills. So is it the substance, or the frequency pattern that works?

Welcome to my world of *innerwise* with many possibilities and many questions.

Okay, enough now with the preliminaries. What do we need for energy treatments?

- The arm-length test for communication
- Sensing, feeling and perceiving—for orientation
- A loving heart
- A testing system that guides and inspires us
- The healing cards, which facilitate the access to the healing frequencies
- The possibility to copy the complete healing symphony to a useable medium, offered by the copy card

- A medium to play back the healing symphony permanently, comparable to an MP3 player: the *innerwise* amulet

The fundamental goal of working with *innerwise* is to create flow—to be in the flow. Certain symptoms may not disappear immediately. "Sprucing up" is not the goal here. My intuition tells me that you have the possibility to change things in your life so that you don't need the symptoms anymore. Sometimes the problems or disorders disappear immediately, and sometimes they take a little longer.

It could also be that you experience some cleansing reactions after your first *innerwise* treatments. If you were blocked for a long time, it's only natural that things have to be cleaned up first: tears, dreams, old images, sweat, loose stools . . . let it all out and away with it!

innerwise®: The Complete Healing System

Contents:
- 309 healing cards
- 6 test cards
- 1 copy card
- 1 amulet
- Booklet with descriptions of all remedies

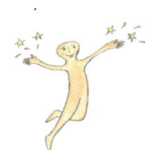

Video clip 7 *innerwise*—an overview

innerwise—an overview

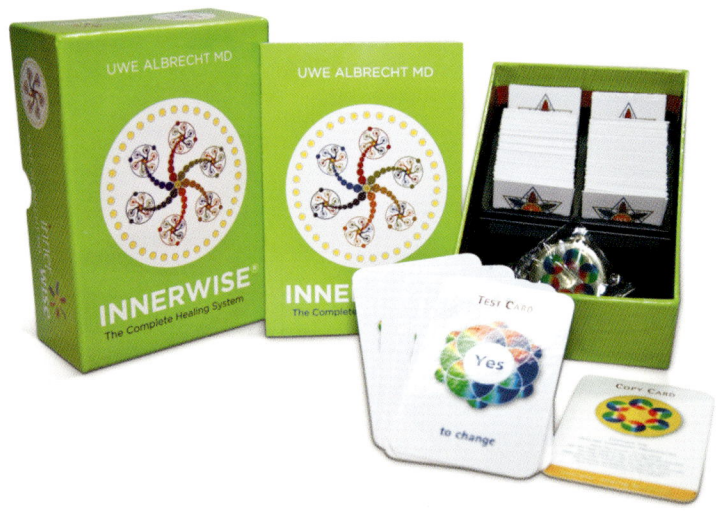

The testing system

If you bring the test cards of *The Complete Healing System* in contact with your body, or take them in your hand, put them into your pocket, or on your belly while lying down, they'll ask you about the topics they contain.

You can also simply look at them and, with the arm-length test, find out what kind of effect they have on you.

If they generate stress—that is, a difference in arm length, you have an issue with one of the card's topics. Each test card contains three topics written on the back, along with individual explanations.

The easiest way to test which one of them generates stress is by putting all six of the test cards in front of you, with the color symbol up.

Since the system has its own intelligence, the test card whose topic should be cleared up first will generate stress first. Another option is to glide your hands over the cards and feel them. One of the test cards will feel different, which will also be the one that generates a difference in arm length. Pick up this card, and your arms will differ in length.

The six test cards: Overview

YES TO CHANGE
I am ready to change.
I am in the now.
I am worth it.

YES TO THE BODY
I nourish myself in healthy ways.
I free myself from poisons.
My body is healthy.

YES TO HONESTY
I am ready to communicate honestly.
I live authentically.
I let go of my compromises.

YES TO LOVE
I love and I am loved.
I love what I was, what I am and what I will be.
I open my heart.

YES TO MYSELF
I am I.
My energy field is clear.
I am happy.

YES TO LIFE
I regain my life energy.
I live my creative potential.
I am in the flow.

The healing cards

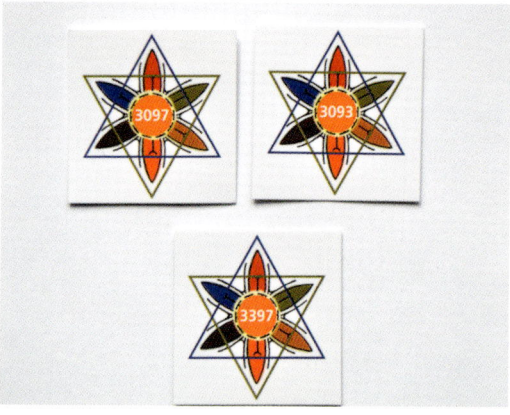

For support, to clear up issues and as a remedy you intuitively draw a healing card and test again. You can then look up the meaning of the cards in the booklet.

Drawing cards intuitively is very easy. Apply spherical vision, concentrate and just reach into the deck—the right card will be in your hand.

You let go of all intentions to control what's happening, and your subconscious has free rein.

If the stress is now completely gone, the cards you drew were the solution. If some residual stress remains, draw another card. On average one to four cards are necessary for each issue.

Maybe you immediately feel that three healing cards are necessary. In this case you draw three at once, though these three cards will almost never lay directly side-by-side. Please don't use a shotgun approach by taking two or three adjacent cards at once; instead, draw them separately.

When you're done with the first test card, put it back and test if a different test card generates stress. If so, this one also needs to be balanced.

The healing cards included in T*he Complete Healing System* from *innerwise* contain the frequencies and energies of:

- Bach flower essences
- Colors
- Animals
- Archangels
- Sounds of celestial bodies
- Schuessler tissue salts
- The signs of the zodiac
- Mary Magdalene soul symbols
- Plants
- Homeopathic remedies
- Crystals

These are just a few of the more than 4,000 *innerwise* frequencies used in the large *innerwise* card system.

Additionally, you have a booklet with simple instructions for use and descriptions of all the healing frequencies.

General advice: The test cards themselves already ask the questions. You don't have to do that in addition; you don't even need to repeat them again in your head.

Once you've had some practice and don't need your attention anymore for the testing itself, you can play freely with the system. You can inquire, deepen, intensify . . . and then you can think about what the answers would mean to you prior to testing.

It's like driving a car—as long as you have to concentrate on the interplay of gears, clutches and gas, it's impossible for you to simultaneously try to find some beautiful music on the car's radio.

After you have balanced all test cards that caused you stress, you may go ahead and ask the test questions related to the daily or weekly health checks described in the annex, followed by your symptoms, or whatever else you want to test. But please be aware that a test card can generate stress not only once, but twice, as it contains several questions, and each time only one topic is activated. (Remember: *innerwise* has its own intelligence!)

Once you've completed your healing symphony (and your arms have replied "No!" to the question: "Is there anything else I can do today?") you copy it to the amulet.

Now you take the amulet in one hand, put the copy card on top of it, and the healing cards in a pile on top of that. The sequence of the cards is of no importance.
Next hold your other hand a few inches above the hand holding the cards.

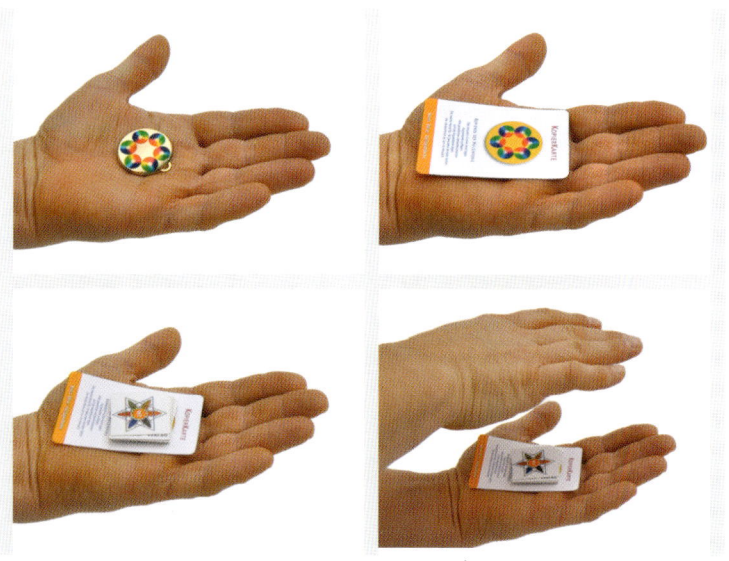

After a few seconds you will notice an energy field building up between your hands. If this field is strong enough, it penetrates through the healing cards, takes on their energies, and transfers them to the amulet. At that moment a vibration wave is generated that tangibly spreads out.

And that's it. Now the healing symphony is contained in the amulet that you can wear around your neck. During the day take it into your hand every once in a while and concentrate on it, maybe do a little meditation with it, as if to say, "Yes, I want to . . .," which intensifies the impact.

You can transfer energies to the amulet multiple times. The next time you work with yourself again, copy the new healing symphony to the amulet. It's neither necessary to cleanse the amulet in-between, nor to delete previous frequencies. You only continue to perceive the healing sounds that resonate with you.

After you've transferred energies to your amulet, it is personalized for you and therefore no longer suitable for other people. There are things in life you don't lend to others, and your *innerwise* amulet is one of them.

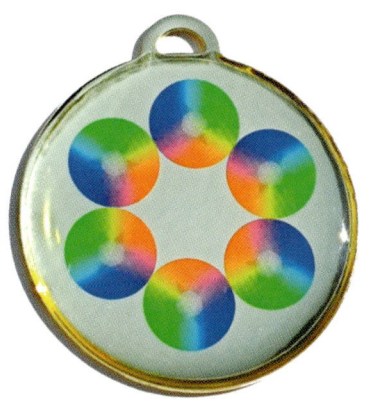

As an inspiration for you, here are a few easy steps you can follow in a treatment:

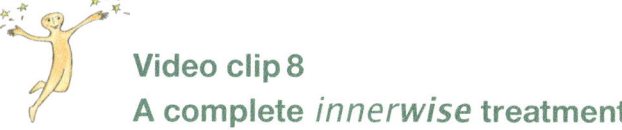

Video clip 8
A complete *innerwise* treatment

You're in a state of rigidity:
Intuitively draw several healing cards until the rigidity is dissolved. A maximum of eight cards may be necessary.

Your arms differ in length when first testing "yes"; they show an initial difference:
Intuitively draw some healing cards until your arms are equally long again. A maximum of five cards may be necessary.

You have a problem or a symptom.
Think of a symptom or a problem that bothers you. This will result in a difference in arm length. Now intuitively draw several cards until the difference is gone. A maximum of ten cards may be necessary.

The daily or weekly check, as described in the annex:
Test all questions and treat the issues that lead to a difference in arm length.

As you can see, you basically always work the same way with the system. Don't forget spherical vision to help you get clear and precise results.

Then you can look up the meaning of the remedies you've selected, since they may hold further important messages for you.

Now you simply put the cards back into the deck, in a random fashion. They're not assorted.

And there is one more thing you need, a vital instrument for treating yourself—trust.

Trust your own intuition.

I've never met a human being who had no intuition, but most people don't trust themselves. Though in reality you have acted intuitively many times before, like the times you fell in love. Even if not everything is made for eternity, it can still be perfect for the moment.

 Tell me Doc, do you have an idea what healing will look like in the future?

It will be fun, playful, and reach deep down to the roots of the problem (without all of that drama, but instead with joy, fun and laughter).

And what do you mean by "future?" The future is now. We're already living it, and whoever wants to continue living in the past can do that as well.

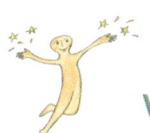 **Video clip 9 Treating a cold**

 And what will become of all the medical doctors?

Don't worry; they're slowly becoming extinct. There're fewer and fewer people who want to practice the old-fashioned way. In British Columbia, Canada, naturopaths only need to take a one-day seminar before they're allowed to write everyday prescriptions because there are no more regular doctors available.

The governments of several German states are already trying to lure medical students with money so that they will open a practice in their part of the country after completing their education.

A revolution in the area of medicine is imminent. And if the doctors don't wake up, the revolution will happen without them. But there's more: A friend of mine owns a big pharmacy in Canada, and right now he's in the process of transforming it into a therapy center. Why? He knows that in a few years time, there'll be no more need for conventional medications. The future belongs to energetic remedies that can be downloaded from a computer. Something that's already possible, and has been used in the Russian space programs for years. This led to several mostly computer-assisted diagnostic and therapeutic devices.

10.

THE BIGGER PICTURE

Human life is like an equation with many variables.
But what are they, and how can they be decoded?

One day in early summer I was sitting in a café in Berlin-Friedrichshafen. A street fair was in full bloom, and a neverending stream of people passed by my table.

How many of those people might be happy, I wondered, and how many still have shining eyes?

I just sat there and looked at the people passing by.

Out of approx. 200 people, only 12 looked genuinely happy, and most of them were children.

Am I expecting too much?

Two months ago I did the same in Vancouver, Canada, where substantially more people looked happy. Does it come down to Germany in general, or just Berlin?

Most people here are marked by life: drooping corners of the mouth; frown wrinkles on their forehead; a resentful expression on their faces; or are not able to look each other in the eyes. They all are energetically empty.

I feel like an alien who is lost and asks himself: "Couldn't God have created more beautiful people?"

For me, only those human beings are beautiful whose soul shines through their eyes.

Having said that, ultimately most people are not really beautiful most of the time, apart from the few happy exceptions.

But wasn't there a time when all human beings were beautiful—right at the beginning of their lives, when they were babies?

It's not important to me how the body looks; the bathroom scale does not decide what is beautiful. Natural beauty comes from inside, from very deep inside.

It requires the existence of at least enough soul so it can still shine. The shining of the soul is creativity that we express, the force of Creation that we live out.

This, of course, leads to many questions:

- Why are so few people happy?
- Why do people allow life to scar them so deeply?
- Why do we hold on to pain for so long?
- Why do partners become more and more alike over the years?
- Why do children so often continue living the patterns of their parents?

I can't find easy answers to these questions, nor can I find easy answers when treating patients and figuring out why they are ill in the first place.

It's all very complex. A + B doesn't equate C, since there're more variables in the equation. The only way to find answers is systemic thinking and working to come closer to the solution.

When I go beyond seeing only the individual (such as by thinking that someone needs a medication for their bellyache) and instead, I really want to understand and heal my patients, I have to see the individual as part of something more complex:

- Them and their family
- Them and their past
- Them and their dreams, desires and the lies they live
- Them and their work

- Them and the environment in which they live, and the picture their environment has of them.
- And if we look at the really big picture: them and the country in which they live. . . .

We need the really big, holistic picture in order to match the details. Only in this way can I as a therapist deliver quality work in these modern times characterized by extremely fast and interconnected lives.

A very simple and beautiful way to become aware of the bigger picture is through imagination or guided meditation—that is, journeys in pictures. This way you'll be able to move freely through time and space. You can analyze "What if?" situations and make energetic connections between people visible.

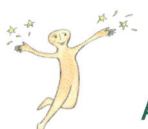

A journey through time

We begin in the present with a few easy exercises:
- How are you?
- How is your stance?
- How do you breathe?
- How is your aura?
- How is your emotional state?
- Do you feel lightness or heaviness?

Now you can embark on your journey through time:
- How did you feel yesterday?
- How did you feel five years ago?
  Travel through time and dive in.

- How did you feel when you were seven years old?
- How did you feel when your mother was three months pregnant with you?

Now come back to the present.

This exercise is much easier when you close your eyes.

Did you notice any differences? It could just be some simple changes at the beginning. Everything is stored inside of us—our bodies haven't forgotten anything.

Everyone can feel it, but most people don't trust themselves.

"Was the slight tension in the shoulder part of it, too?"
"Where does this twinge of sadness come from?"
"What does this sudden heaviness in the feet mean?"

Yes, suddenly there's a twitch, something hurts, the breath changes, you sway while standing, you don't feel well, or suddenly you're happier. . . . It could be all kinds of signs. Trust your perceptions, they're accurate.

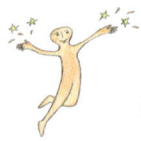 **Remote perception**

Now we go one step further:

Imagine a person you know well but who is not present at this moment.

Now visualize how you become one with this person and can sense inside yourself how this person feels. Notice all changes in you: your breath, stance, spine, emotions and aura.

Now repeat the same exercise with five more people.

You have subconsciously and inadvertently done this exercise countless times. Every time you absorb the energy field of another human being, his or her mood and symptoms also become a part of you.

Now you'll need a break since this work is not that easy.

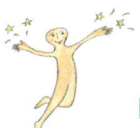

Remote viewing in the past

Now think of one of the individuals in the last exercise, dive in again, and embark on a journey through time:

How did this person feel five days ago, five years ago, when he or she was seven, and during the third month of his or her mother's pregnancy? Then come back again to yourself and the present.

Next embark on another journey through time with another person. In this way, see and feel two or three people in their past.

Now you have done what Jesus has described as compassion: being able to feel what another being feels.

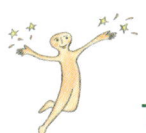

The hand theater

Now we will again go one step further:

Sometimes there are people we prefer not to feel inside ourselves; in this case we use the palm of the hand.

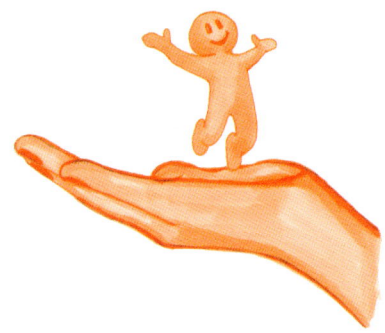

Hold your hand in front of you and open it to receive. Now visualize this person in your hand being about six to ten inches tall. In this way, you can look at him or her from all directions as you do when applying spherical vision. You can see the inner life of these people, if there are energetic connections extending out of or into them, and you can see whether other people are hiding behind them.

A theater in your hand with life itself as the director!

Now you can bring your other hand in front of you and open it to receive. If you want, you can take the same person at another age and then compare the two.

You can also put his or her partner or parents in your second hand and observe the interactions between them.

Ex-partners are always particularly interesting. You can see the energetic links that still exist and are usually invisible—material for countless thrillers! Also the energy-related games that people who are familiar with the dark side of magic play become visible.

Again, this exercise is easiest with your eyes closed.

And in case the person has such negative energy that you don't even want to put him or her in your hand, imagine wearing 100 percent impermeable rubber gloves.

Not only human beings and animals are alive, but also trees, buildings, projects or systems; they all have a history, a soul, and they shape us human beings with their respective energy fields.

These, too, you can perceive using your hand theater, and learn to know and understand them differently.

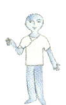
After that much energy work, it's time to go for a walk.

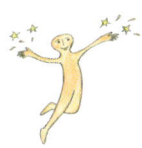
The grass is always greener on the other side, isn't it?

Walk along a street with a row of single houses.

Stop in front of each house, close your eyes and imagine living for at least three years in that house. What is changing in you? How do you feel in each of these houses? Which emotions arise in you? What changes in your body, your stance, your breath . . .?

Yes, what you are feeling is right—houses do carry their own emotions and vibrations. They carry old burdens. Their story and whatever happened in them is often still palpable and has an influence on all the people who live there.

Once you've practiced some more you can continue to also feel gardens and trees.

11.

THE BEST SLEEPER BE THEIR KING

"In Slumberland the most important thing for everybody is sleep. This gave the land its name. But it's not so much a matter of how much or how long they sleep as how well. There is a difference. Someone who sleeps well, so the Slumberlanders say, is kind-hearted and clear-headed. That is why they choose the best sleeper to be their king."

—Michael Ende (edited translation)

Long live the monarchy.

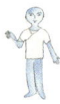

Good morning. Did everybody sleep well?

Don't ask since you know I am a morning grouch. If I didn't know that yesterday not even a tiny sip of beer passed my lips, I would assume it was again one beer too many, because that's exactly how I feel!

Also my back complains every single morning! It keeps telling me: Go get a music video for a morning workout. But when I start to feel better after an hour or so, I always forget about it.

It's like in the film "Groundhog Day": Every evening my back feels great, the body goes to bed, but my head fizzes and bubbles with thoughts and doesn't let me fall asleep. And sure enough, each morning I feel this hangover and backache again.

Please, Doc, help me and test my arms to see what they have to say.

Wow, you really test very gently, feels great.
Look, I can say "yes" and "no," so we can get started.
Okay, I imagine lying in my bed at night. What will you do, arms?

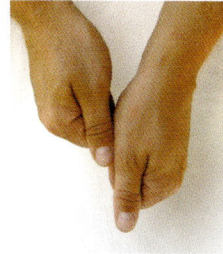

Oh, different length! How surprising! How unpleasant!
  Now let's test how the arms are doing if someone else lies beside or on top of me at night.

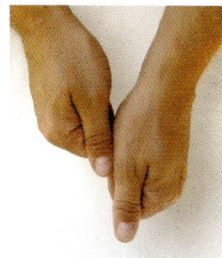

They still differ in length—obviously that is not the solution.

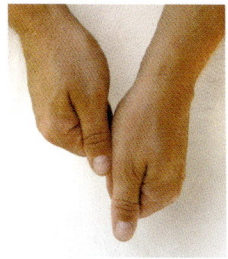

Now let's try another mattress, a really good cold-foam mattress from the land of milk and honey.
  Okay, that's not the solution either.

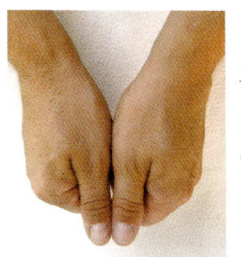

Now I imagine sleeping in another room.
  Oh, interesting, now the thumbs are equally long.

Yes, that was it! I had long planned to move out. Now I can hold the arms responsible when I declare:

"Darling, I will move out, but it wasn't my idea. Instead, I've read this book and now I trust my arms a hundred percent, they're my new guru!"

Today my daughter Hannah is already a blossoming beauty. When I answered her questions and wrote this text for her she was eight years old.

Daddy, I cannot fall asleep.

Daddy, what is a good sleep?

Good sleep means: falling asleep after five to fifteen minutes; sleeping through the night; and after six to seven hours waking up refreshed, with a clear head and without pain and tension in your body.

Anything else is a rotten compromise, induced by electro-smog and geopathology.

Daddy, can you explain this to me?

I'll try. Tell me, how many kids in your class have dark circles under their eyes?

Well, Sophie and Ariane . . . and Jonathan, too, sometimes. But where do they come from Daddy?

They tell us that the person did not sleep well. And they also tell us why: Because all night long you have been charged up with electricity.

And where does the electricity come from, since Sophie and Ariane and Jonathan don't put their fingers into a socket?

There's so much we can't see, hear or smell, but nevertheless it's there. Some people can even feel it. Their body starts to tingle, or they go to bed tired, fall asleep a little, and then wake up startled and can't fall asleep again. You're right, none of them puts their fingers into the socket, but electricity is there anyway. Where do you think the music in the radio comes from?

There are radio masts like the TV tower, and they emit waves or something.

Right, and then the radio turns them into music. The same goes for electricity. There are cables and wires in the walls, extension cords under the bed, plus the cable to the clock radio or the lamp on your nightstand, and they, too, emit something, and we are ourselves the radio receiver. Instead of all the electronics in the radio that are necessary to hear music, we only need water to create electricity in our bodies from the emissions of the cables to produce electricity. We have more than enough of that in our body; three quarters of us is water.

The emissions of the cables are called electromagnetic fields, and if these fields surround us electricity starts to flow through us, because we have all that water in our body. The electricity would not be able to flow through us anymore only if we were as dry as a mummy in the museum. It's like a river—it can only flow if there's water.

Are those fields everywhere?

No, thank goodness. Many people go for a walk in the forest to find some peace and quiet, since there are no electromagnetic fields. We only find them near cables. Thick cables on huge masts can emit these fields very far, whereas the range of the thin cables in our house is only a few feet. But these electromagnetic fields are a bit crazy. Because when there are a few of them they start to play with one another, like children. Sometimes they play "together we are strong," sometimes they take things away from one another, and sometimes they like each other so much that they start to dance together. Therefore, you never know exactly how strong they are at any given moment and place.

Can we measure them?

Yes, with good measuring instruments. But most people don't have those devices.

And what does this electricity do in our body?

If, by chance, we touch a bare power cable, it hurts really badly, and for some people this can get really dangerous. The power those cables emit in form of fields is not as strong, but strong enough to upset our inner clock. We have a clock in our head that tells us if it's currently night or day. And this clock switches different functions in our body on and off. It's called the *pineal gland* or the *third eye* because it contains cells that are sensitive to light, or photosensitive. It functions in our body like the maestro conducting an orchestra. It tells each part what it has to do and sends this information in the form of hormones all through the body.

What are hormones?

When you're sad and I come to you and take you in my arms, caress you and tell you that I love you, and you begin to smile again, then I was your hormone. Hormones deliver messages.

And there is one hormone, called melatonin, which tells you good night when you go to bed, and another hormone that lets you be alert and wide awake when you actively participate in school.

What does electricity do with this hormone melatonin?

The same thing as the Sun. When the Sun shines it is day, and electricity outwits the inner clock, so the body still thinks the Sun is shining (even if it isn't), and so it doesn't produce the hormone that tells you good night, because why should you go to sleep when it's still daylight? Or, imagine that someone puts the wrong notes in front of the maestro, and he then conducts the wrong music.

Many people believe that their day has been so stressful that once in bed, they have to think about everything that happened, and therefore can't fall asleep; or they're lovesick; or somebody they love has left them, or has even died. In these cases one might not be able to really fall asleep for two or three days. But afterward one is so terribly tired that the sleeping pill of the body—melatonin—is enough to fall asleep, even if we're sad or unhappy.

And if it still doesn't work, it's the electricity that makes us believe it's not yet night.

Can you catch the electricity and make it go away?

Of course, we catch the electricity with a cage and send it into the earth. This cage is like a mesh wire shield that you put under your bed and connect to the heating or waterpipe with a cable.

And what if I sleep well, but don't wake up in the morning?

Then you did not really sleep well, and you won't be queen of slumberland. Remember:

Sleeping means falling asleep after five to ten minutes; sleeping through the night; and after six to seven hours waking up refreshed, with a clear head and no pain and tension in your body. Of course, children need more sleep.

Daddy, Jonathan not only has dark circles under his eyes, but he is always restless and fidgety, and he even has to take pills for that. Does this also have to do with electricity?

Yes, but don't tell the company which produces these pills, they will not be happy about that message.

This kind of behavior is called *attention deficit disorder*, ADD. Previously, it was simply known as "hyperactivity," and in the old days these children were called "fidgets." As the name says, the children with hyperactivity are fidgety and can't concentrate. And when the parents or teachers don't know what to do, and their patience is running out, the children have to take these pills.

If these children ate different food, were able to sleep well, learned to relax, their parents saw them as healthy, and—most importantly—the parents could solve their own problems, the children would be totally normal again.

Why should the parents change?

You know, children and parents are very closely connected. When a child comes to me for treatment, I normally treat the parents first, and then the child doesn't really need much treatment anymore. Like sometimes when I'm in a bad mood or stressed, you don't feel so good either.

Imagine if we let you sleep two hours less each night, or let you watch radio and TV constantly, or gave you many sweets, Coke, pudding, sausage and cake to eat, and Mom and Dad are often in a bad mood or stressed out, would you then want to take pills to be happy again?

Oh God, no. That would be really stupid.

I don't think it's so bad that we don't have a TV because I've read many books already.

There's another thing that parents have to change—the belief that their hyperactive child is abnormal. They think their child is ill and the child feels that. It's like if I think and even tell you that you can't do something in the first place. That will not make you feel strong.

Why don't you try to feel how Jonathan might feel: When he gets up in the morning he is still very tired and needs one or two hours until his head is clear. At that time, he has already missed the first class, even if he's physically present. After that, he might be wide awake for two hours and able to concentrate before he gets tired and overwrought again. It's like with little children when the parents have missed their bedtime, and as a result, the children become all hyped-up.

If you were in the same situation as Jonathan, I'm sure you wouldn't have the same good grades you have now.

And that's more or less the whole secret of this ADD or hyperactivity thing.

Sophia's mom always has a backache after she gets up in the morning. Does this also have to do with the electricity?

Not really. Electricity makes the body even more acidic and therefore more sensitive to pain. Instead, it has to do with the place and position of the bed. There are good and bad places to sleep. Wherever cats are cuddling up to sleep is not a good place for human beings. But where dogs, cows, sheep and horses sleep, a human being can sleep well, too.

In the past people referred to earth radiation and water veins for such spots. Today we know that the magnetic field of the Earth contains areas that have positive and negative influences. In addition, there are water veins, faults and lodes.

But the most important ones are the fields of the Earth. They invisibly cover the entire Earth like grids—that's why they're called the Earth's magnetic grids—and every few feet there are spots not suitable for sleeping.

Do they also fool the hormones?

Yes, all cells are fooled at these locations. They're all on alert, and don't communicate with one another; our bodily garbage removal doesn't work anymore either, which makes the body more and more acidic—like streets looking more and more disgusting when the garbage collectors are on strike. And when our body becomes too acidic it hurts and tightens up.

Some people call this a slipped disc, backache or headache, and they suffer and take pills for that.

And why do people not just sleep on spots where their body doesn't become acidic?

Because they don't know any better, or don't want to know. Some people finally get attention when they're ill. Like when you've hurt yourself and we take you in our arms, and immediately the pain diminishes.

Grown-ups also just want someone to hold them in their arms.

And the old knowledge about the good and bad spots has been lost. In the old times priests were initiated in all kinds of knowledge. In old churches they used to play rather ingeniously with these energy fields, and at certain places generated certain states of consciousness.

In Austria even today the use of rods and pendulums to find optimal locations before building a house or digging a well is still widespread.

And for many centuries, in ancient China it was forbidden by imperial decree to build a house before a dowser confirmed that the location was free of harmful energy lines.

And how do I know where there is a good spot for sleeping, if I don't have a cat or a dog?

Why don't you ask your arms? You already know how to do that. Remember, if the arms are equally long, it means "yes," and when they differ in length it means "no," or "stress." Stand relaxed, pull your shoulders forward and let your arms hang loosely at your sides. Now let the thumbs meet. You see; they're equally long. The thumbnails touch exactly at the top. Now say "yes."

Yes.

See, the arms are still equally long. And now say "no."

No. Cool, now their length is different, one hand is longer. That's really a fantastic lie-finder-outer!

Hannah, now imagine that you're lying in your bed. Are your arms equally long, or is there a difference?

Equally long.

Now imagine your bed stands in the corner, and you're lying in it.

Look Daddy, the difference is almost one whole hand.

Why don't you go for a few minutes to the corner and notice how you feel there.

Daddy, my knees are getting wobbly, and I feel weak.

Come back quickly, that's not a good spot. And you see, your arms are telling you this, and you can feel it.

Cool Daddy. Tomorrow I will show this to my friends.

And then you all can be kings and queens of slumberland.

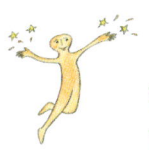

Video clip 10
Test the area where you sleep

12.

Does eating make me ill?

For a while I worked in a fasting clinic. After five days of fasting, no patients there needed medication anymore, never mind if before they took pills for sadness, the heart, their intestines or water retention in their legs.

This was quite a surprise for me as the young doctor I was at the time, since I had just learned for years that certain illnesses led to a kind of lifelong dependency on particular medications and their manufacturers.

Later, I fasted a few times myself, and it was a good experience. I didn't do it to lose weight, but to concentrate on what's important, and for the purpose of purification.

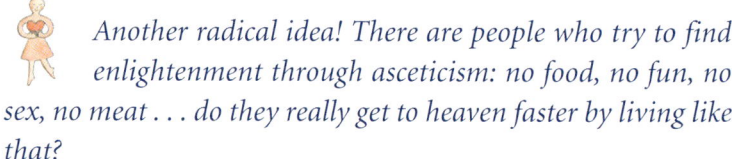

I have a suggestion: From today on, all readers should fast for a period of 10 days.

Another radical idea! There are people who try to find enlightenment through asceticism: no food, no fun, no sex, no meat . . . do they really get to heaven faster by living like that?

Probably, since without joy in their lives they will die sooner.

You both act like an old couple who's constantly arguing; it's starting to get on my nerves.

The reader has bought this book, and the point of this book

is learning how to talk to the body. So let's ask the body what it wants to eat.

 Well, I want chocolate, sugar, ice cream, pudding, vanilla sauce, coffee, beer and lots of meat.

 How egocentric! And the rest of the body has to suffer from your moods.

 What do you mean, suffer? Me, too, I'm a part of the body, and I need my drugs. That small part on the other end of the torso is much smaller than me, and whenever it wants to enjoy his or her lust all others have to comply. Why don't you ask the heart if it's happy when that part down there has a wild go at it? And so often only that lusty area enjoys all the ecstasy, and the rest gets nothing, as usual.

Oftentimes I as the brain feel totally remote-controlled by this little lusty thing down south. So it only seems fair that sometimes I get sugar. It's a fact that I need sugar to work properly—if you don't believe me ask the Doc!

I think we need a supervisor now. Doc, help us please.

Yes, you all want something different: The heart wants to be permanently in love—though the eyes don't want to always be bandaged. The brain wants sugar, and the tissue screams: "Help, an acid storm tide is gathering!"

The intestines want food and need lots of blood in order to digest properly, and the brain says, "Save some of the blood for me, otherwise there'll be a long siesta!"

But seriously, 60 to 70 percent of all human beings don't tolerate certain foods and fall ill with infections of the middle ear, chronic sniffles, asthma, nasal polyps, neurodermatitis, diarrhea or constipation, as well as rheumatism or cellulitis.

Not tolerating something can mean that particular ingredients in the food, especially protein structures, don't agree with them. But it also can mean allergic reactions to something in the food.

When it comes to hay fever, almost everybody believes that it's a reaction to pollen. Though it's actually an allergic reaction to food proteins—they are the real culprits.

You can compare this to not having slept for several nights, and to being totally overwrought and tired as a result. Then somebody comes and caresses you, and you freak out completely. And what's caressing you in the above example is the pollen.

The most frequent intolerance is to cow and chicken protein.

Cow protein is contained in all products made from cow milk. For most human beings it's the first protein foreign to our species that our body is confronted with, and it can be found in almost all baby formulas.

Also residues of bovine protein are injected into our system through vaccines because some vaccines are cultivated in beef broth.

You won't find these facts in the patient information of those vaccines, but I've called a vaccine manufacturer and talked to a friendly female doctor in the production department. When I asked her why I keep finding that vaccines are the cause of allergic reactions to bovine protein, she told me that the vaccine for diphtheria, for example, was cultivated in beef broth. Other vaccines are cultivated in chicken eggs and can cause reactions to chicken protein. Despite all cleaning and purifying, some particles of chicken protein do remain in the vaccine.

And the body does what it's supposed to do when these vaccines are injected—it reacts. But it also reacts to these animal proteins.

The earlier in one's life that the vaccines are injected, the higher the likelihood of often lifelong reactions to these proteins.

If you don't believe this, test the vaccines for tolerance. Have fun!

Some typical signs of intolerance to cow protein are: swellings of all kinds of mucous membranes, sniffles, infections of the middle ear, asthma, cold hands and feet, diarrhea, constipation or belly cramps.

If you want to know now whether you're also intolerant or have negative reactions to these foods, test them:

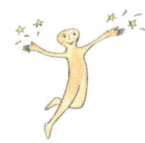

The milk test

Imagine you're eating or drinking the following products: beef, milk, curd, cheese made from cow milk, chocolate with less than 70% cocoa content, dairy ice cream, coffee cream, yoghurt, kefir, buttermilk.

If your power of imagination isn't enough, go to the refrigerator or the nearest supermarket, stand before those products and test them right there and then.

How does your body react? Are the arms still equally long, or do they differ in length? If they're changing in length, test a few more times to be really sure. If the stress, and thus the difference in arms, keeps increasing, it means you are even allergic to those foods.

Now try the same with the following alternative products made from sheep, goat or mare's milk.

These foods often are well tolerated—and voilà, your diet is safe!

Why do we call a swollen up round face a milksop? It's because it shows an allergy to milk and that's why it looks like that.

The familiar reaction to lactose as known from the media and marketing, is really often a reaction to milk protein. But there're no pills for that. Intolerance to milk fat on the other hand is very rare.

But why am I telling you all this? You can find out yourself by testing it.

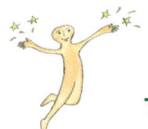

The egg test

Why is it that some people can eat chicken protein only if it's hard-boiled, whereas three-and-a-half-minute eggs make them nauseous? Because they can't tolerate it, and their body tries to tell them.

Chicken protein, which is contained not only in egg whites but also in chicken meat, has a tendency to cause tonsillitis and inflammation in the bowels.

Go and do the arm-length test with egg whites and chicken meat. If you react, you have an official license to eat only the egg yolk. Most people can tolerate that. And turkey becomes the surrogate for chicken.

Though it's possible that your reaction is not to the egg protein but to residues of antibiotics in the meat of chicken raised in intensive poultry farms. This intolerance can show up as pimples the day after you've eaten a meal with chicken.

If you now try to press your belly cheerfully with your hand as deeply as possible, as if you wanted to touch the spine from the front, and if that hurts, your intestines are inflamed. The cause is almost always a reaction to certain foods; in their normal state the intestines don't hurt.

Let's continue a little longer with this kind of self-torture: If you take your thumb and forefinger and pinch a skin fold of your other arm, pressing it hard, it should not hurt either. If it does, it means that too much acid is stored in the tissue. The tissue is swollen with water in order to dilute the acids. And guess what's the most frequent reason for that? That's right, intolerances to certain foods.

Are you up for some practice regarding this topic? Then go and test your entire foods and drinks menu, the content of your refrigerator, and don't forget all the vicarious little satisfactions you nibble on in the evening.

A funny test for children is candy in different colors—the "candy test."

If the arms stay equally long, you tolerate the food. But if they start to differ in length you should avoid them in the future.

If your arms get more and more out of balance when doing further tests, you're allergic to the food. In that case, drop it entirely from your diet.

And don't forget, our food products consist of many ingredients, among them various yummy sweeteners. But thank goodness, these chemicals only cause cancer in the United States; if you eat them in Germany the benevolent hand of the lawmakers, manipulated by lobbyists, protect you (meaning that these chemicals are still allowed here). And unfortunately they still cause cancer.

It's possible that you only have intolerances to one or two ingredients in a particular food. Read the list of ingredients and test the words. And then look for products without these toxins.

When it comes to artificial sweeteners I always think about my dad. He had a potbelly. There came a time when he became diabetic and could no longer put three heaping teaspoons of sugar in his six to ten cups of coffee daily. Instead, he put five sweetener tablets in each cup. By dropping the sugar, he wanted to lower his blood sugar level and hoped to lose weight.

But the body doesn't care if it gets sugar or sweeteners—if it tastes sweet it still triggers the same hormonal reactions. Pavlov and his dog demonstrated that a long time ago. He trained the dog in such a way that the salivating not only began when the dog started to eat, but as soon as he saw the food, and even when the bell sounded simply announcing the food. Therefore, my dad's potbelly got bigger steadily, even without "real" sugar.

Tell me Doc, where do farts actually come from?

Eating half as much is the only sensible way to deal with this. In other words, if you eat a lot, the body can't digest all that food, so it decays slowly and ferments. For instance, when I give a course, I can never eat much, since all day long I need to be totally focused. I simply can't allow myself to give half of the blood that my head needs to the intestines. On those days even a regular meal is too much, and I get gas. And what else could be the reason apart from that? Yes, that's right—intolerance to certain foods, especially milk and chicken protein.

"Fermenting," sounds like something alcoholic. Cheers!

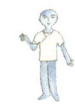
Oh well, it's homebrewed hooch from your own intestines; doesn't make you go blind, but your head will be kind of foggy.

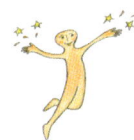
Video clip 11 Going shopping
Going shopping

Hooray, finally we get to go shopping! If you like, go to the nearest supermarket, take the arm-length test and your spherical vision with you and test the products as if you had all the time in the world. Once you find something that you tolerate well and want to buy, you should also test if it's good for the rest of your family.

Remember:
- Always do the pre-test, "yes" and "no!"
- Apply spherical vision.
- Your arms are equally long: You tolerate the product.
- Your arms differ in length: product intolerance
- If you bring your arms together several times in a row regarding a particular product, and the difference in length keeps increasing: You are allergic to the product.

13.

How do I communicate honestly?

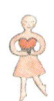 *Why are you such a coward?*

 Are you talking to me? Do you mean me? I'm not a coward! I'm courageous! I have pride; I am intelligent! What else do you wanna hear?

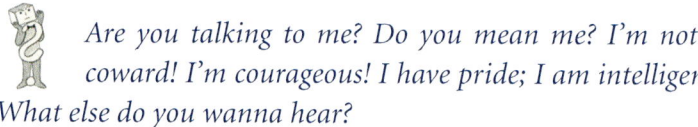 *Your true thoughts. Sorry, but I can't hear them, at least not with my ears.*
Sure, you gabble constantly to yourself, not a minute without inner commentary, but I hear nothing of it coming out of your mouth.
For example, what did you inwardly say to the waitress in the restaurant a minute ago?

 You really want to hear that? I feel embarrassed to say it out loud. Okay, I said: You're cute, your tits are beautiful and I would love to touch them. Still single and available? Do I have the guts to approach you?

 And that was all?

 Oh well, I also commented on her derrière (behind), it's really sexy. And I tried to catch a glimpse from her.

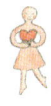   *And what did you say out loud?*

   One cappuccino, please.

   And what did you inwardly say to the man in the blue jacket?

   I can't stand your aggressive voice; those poor children who have to live with you.

   And what did you say out loud?

   Excuse me, may I pass please?

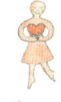   *And what did you excuse yourself for? That you wanted to pass? In what way were you guilty that you had to ask the man for his forgiveness?*

You really are a sorry little man. Living two lives: You don't dare to say what you really think; and then you take the blame for something you never did?

You call that intelligence—knowing when you have to say what?

   Thirteenth chapter—no surprise, there has to be trouble! Though I only practice what I've learned: from my parents, relatives, teachers and the whole of society.

I was a good student and always got excellent grades. I just live like everyone else does, according to the customs of our society.

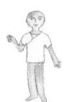 This somehow reminds me of the statement: "It wasn't me, it was Adolf Hitler."

This comparison may seem harsh, but in the past and to this day, there have always existed many societies where most people believed they were doing everything right. They live exactly the way society expects them to. If human beings thought freely, got honest information, listened to their feelings, and oriented themselves on fundamental human values, they would most definitely *not* live that way.

But you now have a rather dangerous tool in your hands, in the truest sense of the word. You have the lie detector. And don't forget spherical vision so the lie detector can function properly.

Listen to the news and test if it's true.

Listen to the different parties' election programs and test which part of their promises they really want to fulfill.

Look at the politicians and test if they really have something to say.

Listen to your own words and test which of them are true.

Big shock! Two-thirds of our worlds are made of lies, and one third of truths.

Our Earth deserves that we as humans grow up and become honest.

When we watch the film "The Invention of Lying" and feel comfortable enough to always speak the absolute truth, then we have made it and are no longer a drag on our great Mother Earth.

Earth and Mars meet. Earth says: "I feel so miserable, I have Homo sapiens." Says Mars: "No problem that will pass."

The meaning of *Homo sapiens* refers to the reasonable, wise, judicious and understanding, diplomatic human.

Since diplomacy is a form of a lie, like any simple lie or statistics, human beings had no choice but to become what they are now. And even the insight into necessities had been arranged. We behave as we have been named: *Nomen est omen.*

The time has come for the *Homo integer*—the integrated human: the honest, pure, decent, intact, whole, sound, unblemished, unspoiled, pristine, authentic, unbroken, complete and incorruptible human. What kind of a world that would be?!

I don't know of a better and shorter description for the intention of this course in healing and the work with **inner-wise**.

How do I communicate honestly, without hurting other people? By using I/WE messages.

Let's try that. Imagine that the day after tomorrow is Christmas, and a visit to your mother-in-law's house is imminent, which results in your children saying: "We don't want to go there." Your partner says: "But it's my mother, we can't disappoint her. We'll only stay a couple of hours." And you already feel miserable at the mere thought of sitting there at the table.

And as if that wasn't bad enough, once at home you get a free bonus—the argument between you and your partner; as a kind of "thank you" for violating your inner Self, so to speak.

Now there are three alternatives to visiting your mother-in-law and not being honest:

1. The fat lie
"We got sick and can't come, SORRY." Some people really get sick then so they have a "real" excuse.

2. Attack and accusation
"You have such bad vibes, and I don't want the children to have to deal with that."

3. Honesty and courage

"We can't come because it's more important for us to spend time together alone."

Our communication is filled with accusations, expectations and patterns. Oftentimes we slap our dialog partner in the face and then wonder why we get an aggressive answer.

"You're the reason that I feel bad."
"You don't care about me anymore!"
"Don't you love me anymore?"
"Your brother would never do such a thing!"
"Pull yourself together, you got to get past that now!"
"We've survived much worse than this!"

"Oh, you're still alive?!" My mother greets me with these words every time I call her, which means the conversation is already finished, as far as I'm concerned. Such phrases can only lead to reactive answers.

What about some "I" messages:

"For me, it is . . ."
"I am feeling . . ."
"We have decided . . ."
"It's good for me to . . ."

This means being and acting like an adult in life and taking responsibility for one's own life, without projection.

How do you best deal with accusations?

Should you receive an aggressive remark from someone, you can defend yourself with answers like: "Yes, but . . ." and partake in the ensuing mudslinging.

Or, you can say "thank you," and clear the energy.

For example: "I hate you." The one-million-dollar answer would then be: "Thank you."

Very simple indeed. This reaction will confuse your counterpart so much that they will run out of steam.

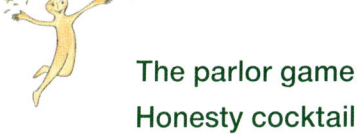

The parlor game:
Honesty cocktail

Next time you're together with some friends and you don't know how to spend an entertaining evening, here is a great game for you. It requires the willingness to take risks, and rest assured you won't forget that evening any time soon. This it how it works:

Ask your partner or your friends for a favor: to be absolutely honest and say what they think of you. And every time, you are only allowed to answer with "thank you," regardless of what they say. After three such statements you change roles.

It's an amusing game, which doesn't require lengthy instructions.

You're not able to tell other people the truth?
Is it cowardice or misguided consideration, because you don't want to hurt him or her?

If you swallow what you want to say, you hurt yourself. You hurt your life energy, your mood and your radiance. Now your stomach, liver, gallbladder and pancreas have to absorb your swallowed hurt, plus your rage, since again you have not told your truth, and that makes them sick.

"My stomach is upset. My blood is up. Something bugs me."—Isn't our language ingenious?

But you don't only hurt yourself, since other people sense

the changes and blame themselves for that: "What in the world have I done wrong, he/she is so different now?"

Great! Due to cowardice, there are now victims on both sides. Whereas a simple cocktail would have been the solution: one-third self-respect, one-third courage, and the rest filled up with honesty—and voilà, it would have been a beautiful encounter!

You could have discovered the other person in a completely new way. You could have seen sides of him or her you'd have never guessed he or she had. But, instead, another bungled opportunity.

And here's another little clue for avoiding bloody noses after drinking honesty cocktails:

Don't slap others in the face if you don't want their fist in your face.

What reaction do you expect if you tell them: "It's your fault that I always have a headache!" You don't really expect understanding, or do you?

Just use "I" messages and use the words "thank you," when in reality you want to say: "Yes, but . . ."

And a few more inspirations:

- "For me, it's better to . . ."
- "We have decided to spend Christmas alone with the children."
- "I'll go and find a new job that challenges and fulfills me more."
- "I thank you for all the experiences we shared, and our time together. Now I will continue on my path alone. . . ."

Do you really think puberty is normal? The kids just have had enough, with all the lies of their elders, teachers and environment.

"I never want to be like that!" and "Your lies make me sick!"—these are the messages of puberty.

There comes a time when kids free themselves from all the lies in order to find out how they want to live their own lives.

Puberty is only normal in a dishonest world. It's the children's outcry for a more honest world.

Being honest doesn't only refer to the words we speak, but to being honest with ourselves and putting an end to compromises. Honesty means authenticity.

What do you want to pass on to your children?

Children will always try to follow our role model. If you live dishonesty in your life, they will do the same.

Set an example as to how you want them to live by living that way yourself. I say this as a father of eight children, with the three oldest who are almost all grown up.

14.

A RELATIONSHIP OR LOVE—
THAT IS THE QUESTION

The rush of falling in love
is often followed by disillusion.
Love changes into a relationship.
Freedom into mutual dependence.
A pretty steep price, isn't it?

 I need you!!!

Thank you to all dogs, cats, children, partners, lovers, flowerpots, parents, chocolates, wines, grandparents, friends and foes—to the entire forest of my life.

The forest
We are like the trees in the forest.
We hold each other.
We need each other.
We share the light.
We protect one another.
We are so happy together.
Our roots are not very strong.
Since we hold on to one another,
they don't have to be strong.
We share the little that we have.

The storm
Me, too, I am life.

The fallen trees
We have become victims of life.

The last tree that is still standing
Alone I am naked and ugly and alone.
Where is everyone??
I am lonely!!!
Help!

The last tree bathed in moonlight
I wished I were beautiful.
I wished I had developed all my abilities.
I wished I wouldn't have always been so considerate
of other people.
I wished I had lived more.
I wished my roots were strong enough to nourish me.
I don't want to be afraid of storms anymore.

Now I have light and can blossom and breathe freely.
Freedom!
I don't have to hide among the masses anymore.

Two beautifully developed trees close to each other
It's a joy to touch you.
We can be alone, we are strong and beautiful,
and we have decided to be a gift to each other.

And should you leave me, I will continue to shine
on my own.

 Mr. Mind, I had no idea you could be so romantic.

Would you prefer if I said it differently? If I was more direct?

 Don't disappoint us; we love your practical style.

 Let's take the word "relationship." A relationship often involves pulling at one another. In German, this "pulling" is even reflected in the equivalent "Beziehung." A real fabulous word—makes you want a lot of that. Sadomasochists first . . .

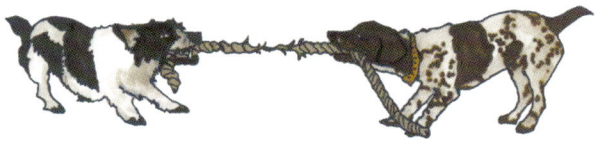

In relationships, we only fill our holes. The physical ones, too, but now I am referring especially to the holes in our souls.

Mr. Mind, you seem to be having a really good day today.

The thing with the holes sounds very interesting. Now it gets rather philosophical my friend. Let's have a closer look at that. Off we go into the depths of the human soul!

 This is how the soul once looked: round, complete and perfect, delicious, simply beautiful to look at. The pie is more than the soul—it also represents love, being connected to the energy of the Source, being whole and complete, as well as trust and health.

Simply perfection.

And then the trouble began.

If, at the moment of conception, you were not wanted by both of your parents ("I'm an accident!"), a trauma occurs, and—*presto*! bam!—the first piece of the pie, or maybe more, is gone.

And in all the years that followed, new shocks and traumas occurred.

The pie got smaller and smaller, as with each trauma, a part of our soul vanishes.

If we look at the soul pie of a typical grown-up specimen of this perfect human race, it looks pretty eaten up. Of the 20 pieces at the beginning, oftentimes only three to five are left.

Now the homunculus is searching for a female or a male. If they then both put together the rest of their pies, it almost looks whole again. If one partner is not enough, mom/dad or a lover may fill in the blank spots.

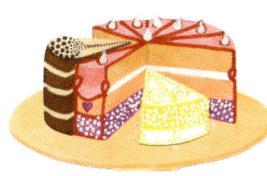

My mother called my father "my better half." Today I finally understand what these words meant. The fact that different kinds of pies come together on a plate only gets apparent later.

Together we are ONE, together we are whole. . . .

Oh man! Only in the beginning of a relationship we utter that kind of nonsense, before we wake up and realize the price we have to pay for this illusion—dependency without limit. Then we can only hope to be strong enough to free ourselves again BEFORE it's too late and love dies.

If the partner completes our own soul pie, the same problems will keep occurring over time. Once one partner takes a self-awareness class, develops him- or herself further and starts healing his or her own pie, a lost piece of the pie returns and fills some of the space that was occupied by his or her "better half." Immediately, this partner doesn't really fit anymore and feels he or she isn't needed any longer, which, in this stage of the relationship, is equated with *not feeling loved anymore*: "Don't you need me anymore?" Or "Don't you love me anymore?"

So the search for someone new begins who might fit better, which can easily turn into a lifelong game.

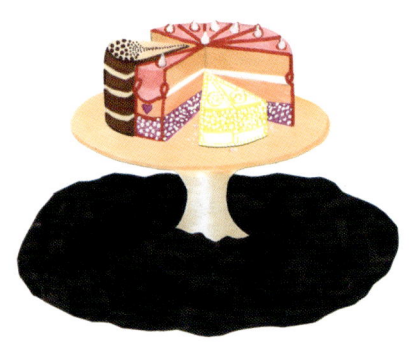

If, through hurt and trauma, more and more pieces of the soul pie disappear, we will more and more often land on the empty plate—a rather slippery affair.
At some point, we will tumble down.

This is how the **pain body** develops—the dark space below the cake plate.

The pain body is the place where we're no longer connected to the energy of the Source; instead, we must try to steal other people's energy through manipulation. The technique most often used for this purpose is the role of the victim, the "poor me," but control, blackmail and aggression are readily used as well.

We're all familiar with this: Situations where we ourselves suck energy, or get sucked dry by someone else. As James Redfield describes it so perfectly in his book *The Celestine Prophecy*; he explains that as human beings we subconsciously tend to control and dominate one another in order to tie someone's energy to us. The other person's energy strengthens us and gives us a feeling of exaltation.

Furthermore, the pain body is the location where trust is replaced by control, and love by a desire to possess. And it's the place where we create all suffering and illness.

Sounds like your regular daily living hell.

"When love first happens, the two individuals are giving each other energy unconsciously and both people feel buoyant and elated. That's the incredible high we all call being 'in love.' Unfortunately, once they expect this feeling to come from the other person, they cut themselves off from the energy in the universe and begin to rely even more on the energy from each other—only now there doesn't seem to be enough and so they stop giving each other energy and fall back into their dramas in an attempt to control each other and force the other's energy their way. At this point the relationship degenerates into the usual power struggle."

—*James Redfield*

The solution?
Making one's own pie whole again, healing one's own soul, thereby not needing the partner any longer and finally loving oneself permanently. And then trying to no longer form a whole sphere out of two halves, but to love each other as two whole spheres.

Here's a test regarding the state of your relationship. Should you currently not have a partner, just remember how it was the last time you had one.

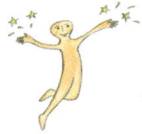

The relationship test

Please mark A, B or C

You can use your conscious mind to find the answers, or make it even more exciting and test them with the arm-length test.

You are my partner; you belong to me.
- A Totally true.
- B Partly true.
- C Not true at all.

If you like me, I also like myself.
- A Totally true.
- B Partly true.
- C Not true at all.

You shall do as I want you to.
- A Totally true.
- B Partly true.
- C Not true at all.

Your processes ruffle and control me.

- ○ A   Totally true.
- ○ B   Partly true.
- ○ C   Not true at all.

You can do many things better than me.

- ○ A   Totally true.
- ○ B   Partly true.
- ○ C   Not true at all.

It's me, always me, who takes responsibility for us.

- ○ A   Totally true.
- ○ B   Partly true.
- ○ C   Not true at all.

Your values are also my values.

- ○ A   Totally true.
- ○ B   Partly true.
- ○ C   Not true at all.

I prefer doing things with you rather than alone or with others.

- ○ A   Totally true.
- ○ B   Partly true.
- ○ C   Not true at all.

I am afraid of your rage.

- ○ A   Totally true.
- ○ B   Partly true.
- ○ C   Not true at all.

I want to protect you from the processes and storms of life.

- ○ A Totally true.
- ○ B Partly true.
- ○ C Not true at all.

Since I've been with you, I've lost touch with more and more friends.

- ○ A Totally true.
- ○ B Partly true.
- ○ C Not true at all.

When I solve your problems, I feel good.

- ○ A Totally true.
- ○ B Partly true.
- ○ C Not true at all.

I am not always honest with you because I don't want to hurt you.

- ○ A Totally true.
- ○ B Partly true.
- ○ C Not true at all.

Even in my dreams I always want to be with only you.

- ○ A Totally true.
- ○ B Partly true.
- ○ C Not true at all.

When you feel bad, I feel bad, too.

- ○ A Totally true.
- ○ B Partly true.
- ○ C Not true at all.

When I can be there for you I feel safe.

- ○ A Totally true.
- ○ B Partly true.
- ○ C Not true at all.

I can't stand it when you suffer.

- ○ A Totally true.
- ○ B Partly true.
- ○ C Not true at all.

I give up my hobbies and interests in order to please you.

- ○ A Totally true.
- ○ B Partly true.
- ○ C Not true at all.

I often ask you whether I should do this or that.

- ○ A Totally true.
- ○ B Partly true.
- ○ C Not true at all.

I am jealous.

- ○ A Totally true.
- ○ B Partly true.
- ○ C Not true at all.

*Your body and sexuality belong to me,
and my body and sexuality belong to you.*

- ○ A   Totally true.
- ○ B   Partly true.
- ○ C   Not true at all.

I can no longer imagine life without you.

- ○ A   Totally true.
- ○ B   Partly true.
- ○ C   Not true at all.

Since I am with you I have changed a lot.

- ○ A   Totally true.
- ○ B   Partly true.
- ○ C   Not true at all.

I ask you what I should wear.

- ○ A   Totally true.
- ○ B   Partly true.
- ○ C   Not true at all.

Evaluation

1. Only A answers:

Sincere condolences. You are nothing; your partner is everything. Your perseverance doesn't give you any bonus points on judgment day, even though your life on Earth is already a living hell.

2. Mostly A und B answers:

You're a good boy/girl. Even though your relationship doesn't make you healthier, at least it's safe. You prefer insurances without risk sharing. You know that in life you have to pay dearly for this.

3. Relatively equal numbers of A, B and C answers:

Dawn on the horizon. You still have some survival instinct left which protects you from the worst. Be more courageous. Every month, one more C. Do you still remember the time when you were still wonderfully excited about each other? Do you want to feel this tingling again? Then go and live C.

4. Almost all C answers:

Keep it up! Your life is going to be worth living. You've almost made it; salvation is near.

5. Only C answers:

You don't need a relationship any more, but you can share your presence with another human being. Now you can really live love.

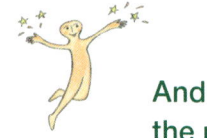

And here you can test the positive version

The statements where you get stress or a "no" response when you test them will be your homework.

Affirmations for a beautiful love relationship

I like myself, even if you don't like it.	○ Yes	○ No
You alone decide for yourself.	○ Yes	○ No
If you don't ask me for help, you can accomplish it alone.	○ Yes	○ No
II am no longer in your shadow.	○ Yes	○ No
You are taken care of, even if I don't do it.	○ Yes	○ No
My values are just my values.	○ Yes	○ No
Your rage belongs only to you; it's not mine.	○ Yes	○ No
I live my truth.	○ Yes	○ No
I protect myself and I know you can protect yourself.	○ Yes	○ No
I respect myself; that way, I feel good.	○ Yes	○ No
Maybe you like my friends, maybe not—I'm going to see them anyway.	○ Yes	○ No

I am worthy of solving my problems myself.	○ Yes	○ No
I am honest with my feelings and thoughts, independent of the consequences.	○ Yes	○ No
Maybe you are in my dreams; maybe you are not.	○ Yes	○ No
I like myself.	○ Yes	○ No
I live my hobbies and interests, with or without you.	○ Yes	○ No
I myself know what is best for me.	○ Yes	○ No
We don't own each other.	○ Yes	○ No
You are grown up and self-responsible, and so am I.	○ Yes	○ No
I give to you, when I truly want to.	○ Yes	○ No
It's my free will to live my sexuality with you.	○ Yes	○ No
It's your free will to live your sexuality with me.	○ Yes	○ No
To live with you is an option in my life.	○ Yes	○ No
I stay true to myself, even if you don't like it.	○ Yes	○ No
I do what's important for me, even if you don't like it.	○ Yes	○ No
All I own is myself, and I am thankful for the time we spend together in this life.	○ Yes	○ No

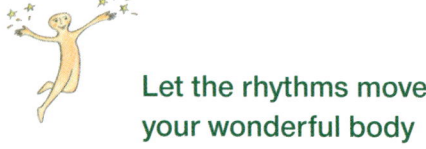

Let the rhythms move your wonderful body

Turn on the music and stand still until you feel where the music begins to vibrate inside of you, resonating with the music. Allow this part of your body to find its own way of moving to the music, and then follow this movement with your entire body. The central beat of your movement always remains the part of your body that responded to the music first.

With the next song, again remain standing still until some part of your body finds its own rhythm.

Different songs will resonate with different parts of your body: pelvis, spine, head, feet . . .

Just observe with amazed eyes.

Now close your eyes and keep dancing.

15.

MINE—YOURS—OURS:
THE PROBLEMS WE SHARE

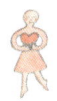 *Tell me sweetheart, aren't you too softhearted at times? Often all your co-suffering with other people is getting on my nerves.*

In those situations my rational mind always says: "Life is what you make of it." But you always want to cry with them.

  Don't be so cruel. After all, you're not a machine. There're people who need help, and I help them.

  Are you also willing to die for another human being?

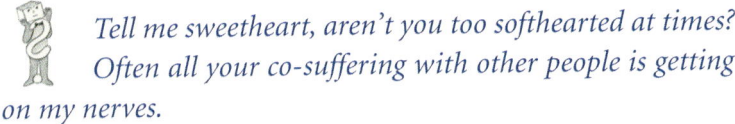 *Now you're going a little too far, after all, I'm not suicidal.*

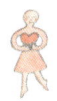 *Oh yes you are. The Doc has found out that at least 30 percent of individuals' illnesses and disorders are not their own, but rather, are being carried for someone else. My problem, your problem, our problem—and in the end, nobody feels responsible to solve it; more specifically, nobody in this mess remembers whose problem it was in the first place.*

And since illness can sometimes lead to death, you are, after all, a suicidal woman.

I am the problem

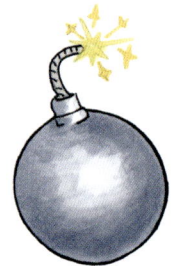

I am the father or the mother of the symptom, so to speak.

If you cultivate me for a while, or if you don't want to notice me, even if I'm there, I will bring forth a symptom.

Now, one should think that everybody hates my guts. After all, I spoil their good and simple lives. I, the big black monster, am ready to explode at any time.

But no, actually, the opposite is true. People even fight over me. They all want to have those problems.

And not only their own, but preferably other people's problems as well.

There is obviously a huge competition among people who can carry the most of me.

And why do you think people do that?

Simply because of love.

Not that they necessarily receive love in return, but they hope to receive it if they sacrifice themselves and keep carrying problems until they crash.

Then, finally, a nurse appears, and memories come back of mommy, the breast, the diapers and the warm comfy uterus. And so the illusion of safety is created.

It's not their problems that make them ill. At least one third of all human beings carry the problems, symptoms, irritations and illnesses of others.

Yes, imagine that: They're crazy enough to act like a hero. Which is true to the old saying "A trouble shared is a trouble halved."

But they don't help the people whose problems they take on, since in reality I am not a problem but a lesson in growth, personalized specifically for each human being.

I am like the breath. After all, it's not possible to breathe, eat or go to the toilet for another person. Everyone has to do that him- or herself. And the same goes for me:

Everybody has to confront me personally; only then is the next step in the game of life possible.

But people sabotage my cause:

Self-sacrifice, suffering vicariously with somebody, total devotion: "I would do anything for you, even die for you"—to whoever may have exalted this idea to be one of the venerable values of society: It was and is wrong. People deprive each other of the right to decide for themselves.

If they don't trust each other to be capable of solving their own problems, to learn their lessons in growth by themselves, they deny each other the opportunity to grow up and take responsibility for their own lives.

They treat the other person like a child whose bottom they have to clean, and in return, they want to get a smile and a kiss.

Over time, this entire spiel has become so perverted that some people with a lot of problems have learned to even use other people to help them carry those problems.

Now the self-sufficient human being, the Homo integer, *enters the stage and shocks everybody with the dictum:*

"I never allow other people to use me, nor do I use other people for my own purposes."

There are some even more radical people who say:

"I never live for other people, nor do I expect others to live for me."

Reading this you may inwardly protest: "But we're meant to be there for each other." When I take care of my small children, I also sacrifice myself for them, give up sleep, going out, freedom.

Children don't want our love and responsibility for them to turn us into victims. Children can sense if we're not feeling well, and they feel responsible for it.

In this way they lose their innocence, since they believe that they're guilty of their parents' problems.

Whereas, in reality, children only want us, as their parents, to serve as an example and inspiration for them, showing them how to live a happy and fulfilled life, while taking our responsibility for them with love and joy.

And that is not total devotion or self-abandonment. If anything, it's the opposite.

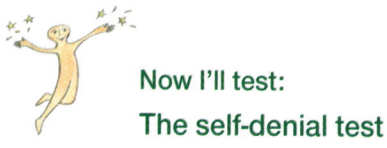

Now I'll test:
The self-denial test

If you get "yes" as an answer, you should take a closer look and find solutions yourself.

I carry . . .% of my total burden for other people.
I let other people carry . . .% of my burden for me.

I allow other people to use me.	○ Yes	○ No
I use other people for myself.	○ Yes	○ No

And here some inspirations regarding remedies

- Speaking the truth
- Writing a letter
- Drawing/painting
- Dancing
- Meditating with crystals
- Using Bach flower essences or homeopathy
- Treating yourself with *The Complete Healing System* from *innerwise*

I carry a burden for	My remedy

16.

BASIC TRAINING: HOW TO BECOME AN ENVIRONMENTAL TOXICOLOGIST

Wherever you are presently—at home, in an airplane or in a vacation home—civilization is already there. And along with civilization come all kinds of chemicals. It's possible that they don't cause you any problems; though it's also possible that they're ruining your health.

Now you're going to be a private detective in your own household, thanks to the basic training as an environmental toxicologist.

You will not stop until your house, your apartment and your room are free of all criminal elements.

They want your life. They want your health. They want your beauty. They're after your energy!

These criminal elements are consciously infiltrated into your household. It's the old idea of the Trojan horse. Shrewd advertisements have made you believe that you can't live without all this crap. Or was it your laziness and lack of attention?

In any case, their last hour has come:

Find these criminal elements with the help of the arm-length test and eliminate them.

Just imagine using these products, and your body will automatically respond: "Good for me." Or, "Don't like it." Or, "Makes me want to puke."

Take a trash can and start with your bathroom.

Test everything using the arm-length test while applying spherical vision.

- Shampoo
- Hair dye
- Hair styling products
- Shower gel
- Soap
- Perfume, deodorant
- Toothpaste
- Make-up
- Shaving products
- . . . and whatever else your find there.

Everything that generates stress, or worse, to which you have an allergic reaction, belongs in the trash can.

Furthermore, you can test the list of ingredients of each product. Just test the words. The worst criminal you will find is the group of parabens: methyl-, ethyl-, propyl- and butylparabens. These chemicals perfectly generate allergic reactions, with extreme itching of the skin, and sometimes can even be found in organic products. Trust only your arms!

Now we come to cleaning agents:

Imagine using them, breathing their scents, getting them on your hands. If you have small children, imagine them putting their fingers into their mouth with all that awful stuff on them.

- Toilet cleaner
- Floor cleaner
- Bathroom cleaner

- Oven cleaner
- Glass cleaner
- Household detergent

And everything that causes stress goes directly into the trash can.

Now let's see what we can find in the kitchen.

Dishwasher tabs whose substances tend to stick to the dish surface, and therefore get into your body next time you eat from this dish. Or do you really believe you can get all the dishes absolutely clean with a few gallons of water?

- Rinse aid
- Dishwashing detergent
- Dishwashing salt
- All spices
- Salt

Back in the sixties, a study was conducted which showed residue of dishwashing detergent in the cells of babies.

Next we go to the laundry room.

Test

- Softeners
- Detergents

The gardeners among us now proceed to the shed.

Test all fertilizers and pesticides to see if those fruits and vegetables are still harmful when ingested.

Test the soil where you intend to plant the vegetables (or where you have already done so).

In a nearby village, single-family homes are being built on the grounds of an old tar factory that has one of the most polluted channels in Europe, with a huge phenol bubble underneath the entire area. This is happening despite the fact that this soil—similar to the Chernobyl region—probably needs a very long time to heal and should therefore not be inhabited by humans. Well then, *bon appétit* to your little ones who enjoy the strawberries and culinary herbs from your garden.

More than once settlements have been built on old garbage dumps with their poisoned soil, and the people who moved there got sick from the toxins.

And for the handymen among you, let's take an excursion to the workshop.

Test which products harm you or your family when using them.

- Wood preservatives
- Paints, lacquers, wood oils . . .

Next we will look at the air in your house.

Close all doors in your home and go outside.

Take a few deep breaths and test if the air generates stress in you.

Now go into the first room, take another deep breath and test the air. In this way, you go from room to room and find the pollution load that stems from wood preservatives, carpets, furniture and paints.

Many years ago, I put a new wall-to-wall wool carpet in one of the rooms in my house. A few days later its smell was so strong that I didn't want to enter the room. Unfortunately, a beautiful orange tree that resided inside the room was not able to flee, so two weeks later it died from the chemical evaporations.

Headaches in attic lofts may be traced back to evaporations of wood preservatives. All of this can be found out by using the air test.

A tip for improving air quality: Get some effective microorganisms (EM). Take a plant humidifier and spray the room/s twice daily with these organisms.

The alternative: Remove the source of the pollutants.

Test the life source of water.

Test your tap water. If it generates stress, boil it and test again. If it continues to generate stress, imagine that you filter the water before drinking it. Here I'm referring to high quality filters only—ones that at a very minimum contain activated carbon cartridges.

You may now test filters that only contain a ceramic inset. I won't tell you the results regarding these filters, you can find out for yourself.

Now you can test all kinds of water processing equipment and systems, as well as all available products for energizing water. You have your own lie detector—use it and find your truth!

Once you are done with your field work as an expert in environmental medicine, think of the people who live with you (if applicable). You can repeat all these tests while imagining that you are that person. Or are they supposed to poison themselves? Or, even better, you can show them how to do the testing themselves.

And now let's throw some light on an important issue.

When my older children were 10, 12 and 14 years old, it was time to inform them. Not about sex, they already knew about that, but about something else that seems to be a part of today's life: drugs. One evening we were having dinner and talked about all the usual drugs: marijuana and hashish, mushrooms, LSD, cocaine, etc.

Afterward, the children tested for themselves which of these substances they would tolerate, and which ones they wouldn't.

The results were clear: Some of these drugs showed no major harmful consequences, while testing revealed an absolute intolerance to others.

As an adult, I can't prevent my children from wanting to try drugs anyway; therefore, I prefer to show them how they can figure out for themselves which substances don't harm them too much. In my practice, I've seen enough people with long-term damages due to drug use.

Using the arm-length test, my children were able to sense and test the effects of these drugs, thereby getting a feeling of how these drugs would affect them.

Hi Doc, are you now going to ask everybody to test drugs?

Yes, absolutely, but if so, you better test ALL drugs: sex, alcohol, chocolate, coffee, medications, tea, jogging releases endogenous morphines), TV, games, etc.

So, the housecleaning is finished.

And in order to keep it so beautifully clean, when shopping you now test if the products in the supermarket are good for you and your family. And you'll never buy anything again that you and your family can't tolerate.

Now we are even going shopping together. You realize that I accompany you in more and more areas of your life. (Just call me your inner wisdom, so there'll be no petty jealousies.)

And now let's go to the supermarket together. . . .

17.

WHO AM I, AND HOW MANY?

If we don't have our own identity, whose life are we living? Not our own, that's for sure.

There are people who are totally clear energetically, and others who are a total energetic chaos. You can feel this the moment you come in contact with them. But what exactly is this chaos? Is it the energy field of another person, or rather his or her own energy field momentarily troubled by an onslaught of tornadoes? Or does a person possibly have more than one energy field? And if there is more than one, where do they come from? Why are they there? What does it mean for the person in question?

In order to prepare yourself for what may be waiting for you in the world of energetic manipulation, I suggest that you reread the books Lord of the Rings *and* Harry Potter. *They will turn out to be more real than you ever dreamed possible.*

Let's assume that a soul has only *one* energy field.

And according to all indications, the turbulences in energetically chaotic people are not tornadoes in their *own* energy field. Therefore, only the alternative remains—external fields affect these people. There is only ONE person, but there are several energy fields. More people than you can imagine have subconsciously allowed that to happen. In my estimate it happens to more than 80 percent of humanity.

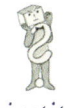 *Are you talking about multiple personalities here, and saying that we should put half the world into a mental institution?*

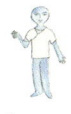 I spent 20 years of my life on one side of a wall. Now everyone can test for him- or herself on which side of the wall the mental institution existed.

As someone who is also interested in science, I've been counting the energy fields of patients for years. And I've found everything, from zero fields up to thousands of fields.

An example: A woman called me very agitatedly demanding an immediate appointment for her husband, saying that it would be a matter of life and death. Her husband is a Buddhist, has a PhD in mathematics, and is presently working as a street cleaner. They went to Thailand together, one year after the tsunami. This man is able to see the souls of the dead, and because of his loving heart, decided to help all those unredeemed souls across the bridge and into the Light so they could find peace. But obviously the souls didn't manage to get across the bridge, and instead ended up in his backpack.

Soon he could hardly walk anymore, and had great difficulties breathing with intense chest pain. When testing what the problem was, it became apparent that his life and heart energy were approaching zero. As if he lay dying under the enormous burden of all those souls.

And the sheer number of those energy fields knocked me over—more than 25,000.

It was hard work to cleanse him of that, but obviously it worked. Two days later I received a happy text message from the couple. They had gone to the beach, and the man felt great again.

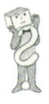 *Hey Doc, why do we burden ourselves with other people's energies?*

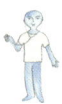 I see two reasons: first, the "helper syndrome," and second, manipulation.

The helper syndrome makes one feel responsible for other people, wanting to help them carry their burden by carrying it together. Oftentimes, the root of this behavior lies way back in the past. These are people who as children were not loved unconditionally, and who now try to gain a kind of substitute love from other people by providing and caring for them.

Manipulation is a different story. People who live in pain use manipulation, they play the role of victim and can only survive through energy vampirism. These people "gift" others with an energetic anchor, if the other allows it. Their goal is to control the other people, thereby draining their energy.

You remember my friend in chapter one who owned the identity of his wife? When he came to see me for a treatment, he had five energy fields. Many people have one to three energy fields. However, only one of these is their own, all others don't belong to them and therefore need to go.

I have another example for a rucksack packed to a bursting point. A pretty hairstylist came to me for a treatment with 500 fields in her backpack. People love to come to her and always feel better afterward. They can talk about their problems, as is often the case when going to the hairdresser. And this good woman always took some of their burden and put it in her own rucksack. One doesn't get a Cross of Merit for this, but perhaps a nice cross on the grave after one's early death instead.

In the meantime she has learned to apply *innerwise* herself and is now able to use her openness and abilities in a positive way, without endangering herself.

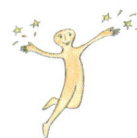

Who am I, and how many?

If you now test, please always do the pre-test first: "yes" and "no" and apply spherical vision, the overview. Look at yourself from outside. Only then will you get honest answers.

	Optimum	My actual state of being	My remedy
I am I			
Number of energy fields throughout my entire being			

Treat yourself immediately, if necessary. Or aren't you curious how it feels to be only with yourself?

 Is Count Dracula still alive? I thought vampires only existed in novels.

 In *The Celestine Prophecy*, James Redfield described the different kinds of manipulation beautifully:

The poor me, playing the victim and thereby generating our sympathy and compassion. This, in turn, generates feelings of guilt in us, and we become reliable energy suppliers for the "poor me."

The aloof forces you to spend a lot of energy to worm the words out of them. It's the old game with the sausage at the end of a stick in front of the dog's nose. It smells delicious, you feel tempted, but in the end, you'll never get it. And when you've lost interest in this sausage, the scent of another unattainable one seduces your nostrils. This, too, is a control drama, and the energy you need to keep the contact going, you deliver straight to the aloof person.

The interrogator will suck you dry with unrelenting criticism: "That was wrong, this is not good enough, are you ever capable of doing anything right? If you had listened to me . . ." Over time you become more and more dependent on such people, since only they know what's right. This criticism has only one purpose: to irritate you so your energy field becomes unstable and free access to your energy is possible. After a relationship like that the first thing you need is fitness training for your self-confidence.

The intimidator threatens you, generates fear in you, and before you know it, he or she owns your energy. You will never have enough energy to fill up such people's energy gap.

(Note: Both sexes can adopt or play out any of these roles.)

**This was a visit with the Frankensteins.
And how do you deal with that?**

1. Is your sense of self-worth strong enough to quit the game?
2. Do you have the courage to address these stupid games, no matter the consequences?
3. Have these games taught you enough so next time you don't get caught in the same dilemma?

Next time you see that the game is being played, say it. Address it; tell the others what it triggers in you. Tell them that through their behavior, you lose your energy, and that you don't want this anymore and will not allow it any longer.

And look closely at where and with whom you yourself play these games.

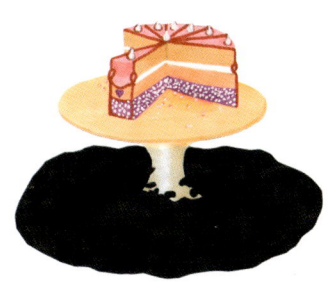

We have to be clear about the fact that all these games are only played because people live from their pain body. They've been kicked off the pie plate of their soul. And with that, they've lost their connection to the Divine, to love, to energy. So the only possibility they have to survive is to rob others of *their* energy.

The fact that we can understand their behavior must not mislead us to release them from their responsibility to connect themselves again with their own energy source. And the first step is realizing that this game is played after all.

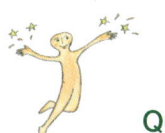
Quit the game

Make a list of the 3 people
who draw the most energy FROM YOU:

1. _____
2. _____
3. _____

Make a list of the 3 people
YOU draw the most energy from:

1. _____
2. _____
3. _____

Now you can write six letters, or e-mails, have six phone conversations or look into six pairs of eyes, and end once and for all the stealing of energy.

But remember: without accusations and without thrusting a fist into someone's face. Speak in "I" messages, from your heart.

For instance: "Finally I understand that I rob you of your energy with my behavior. I don't want to do this anymore and ask for your help: Please tell me honestly any time I behave like that again, especially if I don't realize it. Thank you."

Or: "I don't feel good when I am with you. My energy drops, and my mood sinks. This gives me the feeling that I'm not good. I've decided not to accept this anymore. I like you, but when we are on the same level."

A few more words in regard to the energetic world.

The energetic world is also a world of duality. This means that not everything there is good and loving.

Not every therapist working with energy generates good results, not every initiation is for the good of the person concerned.

Sadly, the majority of therapists working with energy are not "clean," but accompanied by energies from the other side, which they pass on to their clients. The reasons for this are the fear, power and control issues of these therapists. One could use the term "possession" here—for me personally, this term is too narrow in regard to its meaning; it doesn't point out the personal responsibility.

When I test the number of my own energy fields or those of others, and find more than one, I always know that something is not okay. These energy fields can have a variety of traits, all the way to characteristics of the gravest possession. But they can also be very sweet, though this is quite rare.

Pregnant women have two energy fields. Of course, the one of the child is always present as a second field.

For years a patient of mine heard a voice that guided him, gave him instructions and lots of power, energy and wealth. He paid for this with a lot of pain. I told him to ask the voice who it was. To which the voice replied: "I am God, your Father. I am the pure spirit."

When I dared to question this, the voice belted out its commentary: "F—ck you, f—ck you, f—ck you, I'm gonna get you, too!"

(So much for the spirit that wanted us to believe he was pure and a God incarnate.)

The sources that become accessible for us in the energetic world also have qualities like light and shadow, good and bad, day and night. These qualities don't only exist on the human level, but also on the higher energetic levels.

According to Burkhard Heim, there are 12 world dimensions, and he called the upper four "GOK—God only knows."*
He was able to outline all levels mathematically, but for those four he wasn't able to describe their function. I would call these four levels divine and pure; everything lower is not, because it's caught in duality, carrying light and shadow.

---

*Translaters note: In German: GAB (Gott allein bekannt)

Besides, it's of no importance if we call it God, Source, Creation, the Absolute . . .

The One can only experience itself through duality. How could we understand the concept of time if day and night did not exist?

 So God created light and shadow to dispel his eternal boredom?

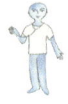 There are many people who call themselves pure channels: "The angels talk to me." Though all these people's farts stink exactly like the farts of everyone else.

There are many energy therapies, spiritual schools, and especially the old guru systems, that use energies unchecked and pass them on. Many of these therapies use manipulation and try to get the most precious quality we human beings possess—our heart energy. Cults and sects of all kinds are also hot for this light and want to use it for their own purposes. Then, the old fairy tale about the cold heart suddenly becomes reality.

Ron Smothermon commented on this in *The Man-Woman Book*: "Real enlightenment is simple and easy to understand. That guru hocus-pocus will give you problems, however."

There's a simple and easy way for you to test if someone is energetically clean and without manipulative intentions, and if you should embark on energy work with this person, getting involved in certain therapies, Reiki, family constellation work, initiations, etc. after etc.

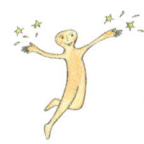

Five questions for testing therapists and spiritual teachers

- Does this person have his or her own soul identity (I am I)?
- Does this person have more than one energy field?
- Is this person free of manipulation?
- Does this person work for the highest good of everyone?
- Is love this person's basic motivation?

For testing therapy systems and spiritual institutions, I recommend the following statement:

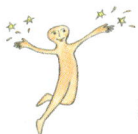

Statement for testing systems

All present energies serve solely human growth, are based on the power of love, and free of energy vampirism and manipulation.

If you get a "no" as a response to any of these questions, look for someone else, another path, or even better: help yourself.

18.

HEALING THE "SOUL PIE"

*The retrieval of parts of the soul lost due
to deep hurt is the key to healing.*

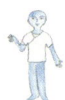 Christmas was almost there, and again I was about to lose a child.

I could not feel my little daughter anymore. I played with her, fed her, cuddled her, tucked her in at night, but she was almost a stranger to me, as if she was not my own child.

By now she was nearly two years old, and her short life until now had not been easy. Don't misunderstand me; she was not ill. But her soul had almost vanished.

My heart couldn't feel her anymore. There's hardly anything worse for parents than not being able to feel their own children.

She was already with us half a year before she was conceived. She sat on my shoulder, flew away again, and came back in my dreams. She had just waited for the perfect moment to acquire a body.

But it looked as though that wasn't possible anymore. The relationship between my partner and me was seriously on the rocks, one acid test after another. But the little soul had chosen us as her parents, her sister (who was just two years old) and her older siblings. Thanks to her own strength, she used one of the few chances that presented themselves to her.

Her mother was overwhelmed with this situation; she had already begun to walk her life path separate from mine.

At the last moment, a friend recommended a book about the emotional consequences of abortion, which arrived just three days prior to the appointed time for the termination of pregnancy.

So the little soul had overcome another hurdle. But this time, again, for a high price, as I later learned.

For the rest of the pregnancy, the little soul and I were allowed to learn how to stay connected with each other despite the distance. I was forbidden to touch the mother's belly.

I remembered my grandmother in Germany who hadn't heard from my grandfather for years after he had been a prisoner of war in Siberia. Even messages about his alleged death could not interrupt the connection between the two of them. My grandmother simply knew that he was alive. She felt it in her heart. And she had a wonderful heart.

Eventually he returned, and they lived together up to a blessed old age.

When our little girl was three months old, her mother took her and her sister and moved out, and the physical distance between us got even bigger.

Oftentimes when mothers are exhausted, this gives fathers a chance, especially when the children have been used as pawns in order to hurt the other.

And that's exactly what happened. It didn't take too long before I was allowed to see my daughters again and have them spend the night in my house. Slowly we established a kind of regularity in our lives, and the children spent half of the time with me.

I was happy—my daughters were back again.

But something was not right. I realized that I could feel my little daughter less and less; she became so much like a stranger to me that I almost reached the point of giving up.

I had no problem feeling my other daughter who was two

years older, which meant that my heart was not yet cold. But what then was the reason? I felt desperate; all my therapeutic abilities didn't help.

Then, one day, I saw a movie in which Alberto Villoldo talked about soul retrieval of the ancient Incas.

That was it!

With each hurt or trauma children lose a part of their soul.

So my little daughter had in fact mastered all hurdles, but for a price: There was almost nothing left of her soul.

When we talk about love, we actually mean that through the soul of another person we're able to touch and feel the Divine.

As I was allowed to observe later with my patients, oftentimes this loss of the soul already begins at the moment of conception.

In workshops I requested the participants to draw their soul pie. A complete pie means that all parts of the soul are there and can be lived.

Sadly, the drawings exceeded all my worst expectations.

Starting with the idea of 20 wedges for a complete pie, most had only one to six pieces left on their plate. In addition, some had pieces of pies from their partners and ex-partners on their plate (more on this later).

Are we really such soul cripples? How can I say that I live my soul's plan when my soul is notably absent?

And when I realize this what shall I do? Can one get back all those lost years?

The shamans of the Incas could. For them, it was always an important task to keep the soul of each child whole and retrieve lost parts if necessary.

Since I had no shamanistic training, I tried to do the same with my little daughter by using the techniques I had developed.

I remembered her soul when she was still an angel and we met each other for the first time. She was breathtakingly beautiful and perfect.

So one night when she was asleep, I sat down beside her and began to meditate. I invited all parts of her soul that were not present at that moment. It was a simultaneously sad and happy moment, so many memories came back again, including all those that had been hidden.

And then my heart opened, and the little child in front of me was again my daughter. I could feel her again, my body and my soul vibrated with happiness—it felt like a miracle. My daughter, who I had almost lost, was sleeping peacefully before my eyes, beauty and purity incarnate. She woke up, and I took her in my arms.

Those two difficult years had given me a huge gift, one that I could use from now on to help other people as well.

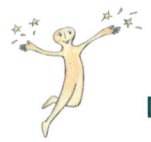

Draw your soul pie

To begin, you should get a sense of how it felt when your soul pie was whole and perfect. To do this, you have to go far back, before the first hurt in your life, (and just to be sure go back to the moment even before your conception). That's how your soul pie once looked.

Now you can draw the present state.

Draw a circle and from there, sketch which soul fragments are still present.

Don't think about it, just sit down and start drawing intuitively.

How much of your soul's completeness is left?

Maybe your pie doesn't have a center or has suffered corrosion; possibly some residual lumps are scattered around, or entire pieces are missing.

Or, it may be that you want to draw individual pieces with another pencil, another color.

Those would be the parts that other people borrowed from you.

You can also test it:
How much of your soul is currently present in percents?

Of my initially complete soul, . . .% is currently present.

Ask your arms. The answer will be somewhere between 0 and 100 percent.

There is no need to be frustrated if the percentage is not very high; even 20 percent is pretty good.

You don't have to prove anything to anyone. You do this test only for yourself, and please don't forget spherical vision: Look at yourself from outside and from all directions.

In one of the next acts of this drama I'll show you how you can heal your soul again.

After 18 years of: developing energy therapy systems; self-awareness; emotional work; studying different wisdom teachings; teaching; eight children; four marriages; four further relationships; involuntary dealing with gurus and other spiritual power systems (due to my partners); and moments when I didn't want to go on, but always made a fresh start, it has finally happened—I've experienced what it means to be healed.

Here an excerpt from my journal:

It's late evening, and I'm sitting in my—let's say uncluttered, my children call it empty—living room and laugh about my life.

I laugh about all the drama, the pain, all the experiences and exciting moments.

I feel as if I am looking back upon my life after death, finally able to see the whole picture, and I realize with delight how it has all been created perfectly so that I could enjoy the wealth of experiences.

Now I feel what happiness really is.

Happiness as a state of Being, and not only as a moment in time.

I am free.

19.

DO I TOLERATE MY DENTAL MATERIALS, VITAMINS AND MEDICATIONS?

Or are they even harmful for me?
How can I find out if I need these remedies?

Hey Doc, did Pippi Longstocking puff your face up yesterday and paint red spots on it?

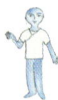
How embarrassing. I am co-author of a book like this one, and then this happens.

Come on now; don't be shy, what happened?

I went to my dentist because one of my teeth needed a new crown. And since it had to be customized, she gave me a temporary crown so the teeth wouldn't move due to a difference in height.

Before the treatment, we tested all the materials needed: the anesthetic, the lining, the material for the crown; there was only one thing we didn't test: the composite resin for the temporary crown.

Four days later my entire body was itching and started to puff up. I felt as if I had swallowed a whole month worth of contraception pills, and my body believed to be pregnant and quickly decided to store a few gallons of water. I immediately removed the temporary crown, and now I almost look normal again. And the itching has stopped, too.

So much for being authentic and living what you preach.

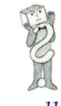 *Considering that you're authentic, everybody will have a laugh just by looking at you. That finally makes you really human.*

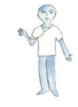 I quickly had the opportunity to put this experience into practice; today a patient came to me who suffers from neurodermatitis.

She had already come to see me once before, about a year ago. At that time we used the arm-length test to find out that she was allergic to amalgam and the composite material in her teeth. Then she went to have those materials removed and her skin healed. This time she came back because her skin had started to itch again. It turned out that her dentist had filled a new hole in her tooth again with the same composite material.

Now she has to go back to her dentist in order to remove all composite resin, and her skin will heal without her having to use any kind of cream. As the old saying goes: "Natural beauty comes from within." And our skin is the organ that yells: "Hello, something is really wrong here!"

Our skin surely doesn't say: "Please rub me with cortisone cream and gag me." Only dermatologists, who can't think out of the box and who don't find out (like a clever detective) why the skin is reacting in this way, say that.

And you know what happens when the skin can't scream for help anymore due to all the cortisone cream? The body pushes the problem one level deeper, and the lungs or intestines begin to react and get sick. As they used to say in ancient China (and rightly so): The skin is the opening organ of the meridian pair lungs and large intestine.

A few years ago I was asked to treat Frederic. He was 17 years old and spending his life lying immobile in a nursing home; he was the only youngster among old people. Only with great pain and in slow motion was he able to move a little; he needed to be fed and had bowel movements only every seven to ten days. His entire body was poisoned.

Six months later Frederic could go out dancing and flirting with girls again.

I had helped him to release toxins and restore energy flows. The troubled organs were able to regenerate themselves.

The solution to the riddle: It all began when Frederic was 14 years old. At that time he played a lot of sports and was always very hungry afterward. So each day he consumed one to two cans of tuna. He didn't know that he was allergic to mercury, which is stored in great amounts in tuna. Within two years, he wound up in a nursing home for permanent and hospice care, because at some point, the doctors in the hospitals had given up on him.

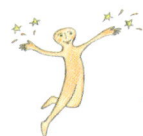

Testing your dental materials

And now the moment of truth has come for you:

Please do again the pre-test and see if you can say "yes" or "no," and don't forget to use spherical vision during the testing.

If you have fillings in your teeth, touch one filling after the other with your tongue and simultaneously test using your arms to see if you have reactions to the fillings. If there is a reaction in arm-length, stay with your tongue on that particular tooth and test three more times. If you test several times consecutively and the difference in length grows, you are allergic to the material. Bingo!

Video clip 12 Dental test

Teeth		Teeth	
First quadrant (upper right)	Second quadrant (upper left)	First quadrant (upper right)	Second quadrant (upper left)
18 17 16 15 14 13 12 11	21 22 23 24 25 26 27 28	1 2 3 4 5 6 7 8	9 10 11 12 13 14 15 16
48 47 46 45 44 43 42 41	31 32 33 34 35 36 37 38	32 31 30 29 28 27 26 25	24 23 22 21 20 19 18 17
Fourth quadrant (lower right)	Third quadrant (lower left)	Fourth quadrant (lower right)	Third quadrant (lower left)
Europe		Amerika	

Should you have anything artificial somewhere else in your body, for instance a device in your uterus, rings in your navel, tar in your lungs, contact lenses in your eyes, medications in your blood, pills for happiness in your brain, think of those and test them, too.

If you have an allergic reaction to one or all of those materials, you have a choice: Either you continue suffering from them, and you wilt prematurely, or you remove them from your body. You should never take anything or have anything implanted in your body to which you have an allergic reaction. An absolute NO GO!!

Now you might have a problem: How can you persuade your dentist to believe your arms? And how can you cope with the professional pride of your doctor? How can a non-doctor know something better than a doctor?

The solution:

- A therapist serves people, not the other way around.
- The time for authoritarian systems is over, even if many doctors have not realized that yet.

- Very simple, show them the arm-length test.
- Should that not suffice say: "Thank you and good-bye!"
- Time to look for a new doctor or therapist.
  If many of us act accordingly, the days of those diehards are seriously numbered.

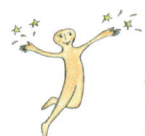 Okay, we're done with the teeth, now let's turn to vitamins and other nutritional supplements. Test these, too. They may or may not generate stress, or you may be allergic to them. And even if you tolerate them, the question remains about whether or not you need them. You don't need to take anything your body doesn't need. And all of this information can be entered in the following chart:

Test for yourself vitamins, medications, etc.

Nutritional supplements & vitamins	Stress	No stress	Allergy	I need it	I don't need it

Now the moment of truth for your medications has come. Please don't forget oral contraceptives and homeopathic remedies. . . .

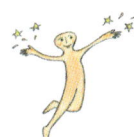

Video clip 13 Testing vaccinations

Medications	Stress	No stress	Allergy	I need it	I don't need it

Please always test all five questions since it's possible you don't tolerate something, but need it anyhow.

 And now we come to a slightly more complicated subject:

If you don't tolerate a medicine or even have an allergic reaction, you can't simply discontinue it. In this case you need a therapist or doctor who supports you.

Some remedies must be reduced gradually, while others have to be substituted.

My last statements are not only for legal reasons, but also based on many years of experience that have taught me that some drug withdrawals need support. Don't immediately object to the term "drug," since according to the World Health Organization (WHO) each active agent capable of changing functions in a living organism without being a food item constitutes a drug.

And sometimes we have to live with the fact that medications generate stress because currently there are no other solutions available. However, if you have an allergic reaction to a medication you and your doctor have to find an alternative. Otherwise the medication destroys you more than it benefits you.

At least you can test what reduces or balances the stress. This can be herbs, vitamins or homeopathic remedies. Or you find something in *The Complete Healing System* from **innerwise**. Conventional medicine does this same practice, they often combine a medication with gastric protection so the stomach doesn't suffer from corrosion.

So off you go to your doctor, and put the facts on the table:

"Dear doctor, since I am taking your pill for high hypertension the pressure is indeed down, but my wiener is, too, and that's unacceptable!"

The female version for this statement would be: ". . . my mood stays down, too. Not acceptable."

Put the note with the side effects on the doctor's desk, explain the arm-length test (a bit of tutoring for your doc about neurological reflexes) and request a different solution. Or do you prefer to continue being a guinea pig?

Modern Western medicine thinks in the form of statistical probabilities. But we humans are not statistical probabilities; each of us is a unique reality.

Medicine makes you believe that if at some point you needed blood pressure medication you would need to take it for the rest of your life. And most people believe this nonsense.

With hypertension the pressure in your entire body is too high: in your head, your vessels, your chest . . . you're under pressure.

Change your life so the pressure can disappear. Open your breathing so you can once again breathe deeply in and out, and give yourself a full treatment. Oftentimes, that's enough. Now you need a blood pressure monitor so you can measure the pressure and see when it sinks, and when you and your doctor agree you can reduce the medication or discontinue it completely.

Once a woman patient came to me who suffered from severe depression. Three weeks earlier her job had caused her extreme stress, and she had a singular high blood pressure reading. Her doctor immediately prescribed the maximum program, with three medications to be taken daily. She didn't tolerate two of these medications at all. Without searching for the cause of this intolerance, or doing any long-term measurements of the blood pressure, he utilized his own position of power and said: "From now on you have to take these medications as long as you live." No! We managed to change this "lifelong sentence" into a week. Today she is well again, able to deal with and resolve her issues, and the long-term measurement shows a normal blood pressure reading.

In about 80 percent of all cases, patients are able to discard the medications at some point.

And the ability to free yourself from taking medication is not only true for high blood pressure: If you suffer from type 2 diabetes, I suggest you read Michael Montignac's book *Dine Out and Lose Weight*. The author describes the best alternatives. With a fasting cure the blood sugar returns to normal in less than a week.

Depression: The translation for this word means "degradation." Of what? Of life energy, and that is something you can get back. You only have to master the small task of ending all compromises that take away your energy.

And we could continue to look at many illnesses in this manner. In the end, there always remains the one key to healing: Change your life!

In the eyes of most people this seems impossible, so they continue to need pills.

Every human being is allowed to suffer as long as it's necessary for him or her to learn something.

20.

THE DIVINE STOCKPOT

*What if there are no past lives, and our souls
don't continue to exist after we die?*

Some believe in hell, others in heaven, after we die; atheists only believe in dust, Hindus believe in karma, and modern esoteric people believe in reincarnation.

I have no clue which of these beliefs is really true, but one day we will all experience it.

My father was a philosopher and encouraged me to think about things. It's in this spirit that I would like to invite you to reflect on these concepts in terms of thesis and antithesis.

Karma, past lives and so on—are they really what we think they are?

Through past-life regression, we can gain access to our past lives:

- when we used to live,
- who we used to be,
- where and how we incurred guilt,
- what we didn't do because we were too cowardly,
- and with whom we shared various experiences.

Then, we can attempt to clear up some karmic charges; or at least, we'll have good excuses for bad behavior in this life.

As you continue reading, chances are you'll find that you can't use these excuses any longer. You may find that knowing how saintly or royal you were in a past life doesn't make your behavior in this life any more noble. Then even the statement: "I think we met in a past life" may actually be no more than a way of hitting on someone.

So . . . what if there was no individual karma?

Instead, what if we offered all individual experiences to the One after we died and let them go completely?

The meaning of our human existence would then only consist of having experiences on all levels—physical, mental, energetic, emotional and spiritual.

These experiences and maturation make up our true fortune, not the wealth we accumulate while on Earth.

And who said that life on Earth was always going to be nice and easy? Pain, fear and loss are as much a part of life and learning as happiness and abundance are.

If you now think of all you've lost and experienced, all your feelings of guilt or negative experiences, you can leave your victim role behind and tell yourself: "I've become rich—rich in experiences." And since we can't hold on to anything, it's likely that we also lose these riches when we die.

When we're back in the Light, we're free from all human burdens. And when we're back in the Light, we're an integral part of it, not an energy-saving lamp. There, our human suffering doesn't exist; there's no pain. In the Light, we can recover and prepare for the next journey.

In this Light, everyone is equal: the prostitute, the pope, the atheist, the Satanist, the homeless person, the millionaire, the murderer—everyone, without exception.

Those who believe in hell will have to wait until their next incarnation on Earth in order to re-create it anew for themselves.

In the Light, we are perfect and complete, one with everything. We are free.

We are like a drop of water that after death returns to the great water and becomes part of it. This drop of water never existed in this exact consistency before, and will never exist in that form in the future.

We will again become one with ALL THAT IS, and all that is individual dissolves. This includes the past, the future and even the soul itself.

Of course, you can refer to ALL THAT IS by a different name, such as the great water, the Light, God or Allah. Everyone according to his or her own preference.

When another drop separates from the great water, this separation from ALL THAT IS again turns it into something individual, and a new soul is born.

It's as if ALL THAT IS took a break from itself and went on an adventure to once more go for the full experience.

As a newly created individual, still completely pure and innocent, we then proceed to the divine stockpot, which contains the experiences and lessons of all human beings who ever lived.

From there, we then take a big ladle for our personal bowl. Some people who are very hungry for life seem to take a particularly large scoop, or even two.

The stockpot is like a secondhand store where every soul has to find the right clothes. Thus, the stock bowl contains the tasks and contracts for *this* life—that is, roughly the circumstances, a new name, a new face and a new past.

Sounds like a witness-protection program.

It thereby holds the basic energetic charges that we bring into this life. Since it's composed of the experiences of numerous people, we're able to remember different aspects and times and carry the charges of many others within us.

This means that our soul doesn't drag around specific karma forever.

Our soul hasn't experienced the past belonging to the new identity, but we have absorbed it with the stock.

We're not a special soul, nor are we a particularly old, wise or even young and inexperienced one—there is no incarnation of a special person. Rather, we're just a part of the Light that has to eat the stock it has brewed—that is, face the music.

Even though Cleopatra *did* once exist, you may confidently stop believing that you are her reincarnation, but of course, if you learned this during a past-life regression, your ego is probably getting a real kick out of it.

It won't make wrinkles and love handles look any sexier, though.

Thus, I say good-bye to any karmic excuses or pretexts, to spiritual vanity, to living in the past and to all forms of spiritual classification systems.

Welcome to a world where you're responsible for everything you experience here on Earth.
You are the creator of your own reality.

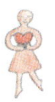
Here comes the grand motto of the day:
Death is the fastest way to enlightenment, but life can be the greatest way to enjoy enlightenment.

Wow, today everyone is going crazy with intelligence and inspiration!

Your father must have been a smart and noble man, especially if we get so many gifts thanks to him.

In addition, he was unique, there was never anyone like him before, and there will never be anyone like him again.

 To how many gurus and belief systems do we give the power to determine our thoughts, emotions and deeds?

Which truths should we accept as irrefutable, and which not?

These were my inspirations:

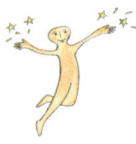 **Simply test your own truth using the arm-length test and spherical vision**

Is karma a reality?	○ Yes ○ No
Have you lived before as your present soul?	○ Yes ○ No

21.

HEALING THE PAST

Now you know a little more about me and my way of thinking. You've become a bit hardier, more accustomed to it, which is good because you'll need to be now.

Test with your arms if you can get a "yes" and a "no."
Remember: Always do the pre-test.
Now, imagine your parents are making love and conceive you.
Test with your arms if this idea causes you stress.
Is it a bit of stress or great stress?
Now imagine your mother conceiving you. Stress, yes or no?
And now your father. Stress, yes or no?

At this point a few lights might dawn upon you, and you may begin to understand why your heart connection to your parents might be or possibly used to be let's say "interesting," and why your connection to each of them might feel very different.

From my experience I would suggest that you DO NOT try to completely feel this incidence of conception again, since there's the possibility that impressions and thoughts will get stuck in your head.

Now let's continue with your life:

Imagine you're in your mother's womb. Do you feel stress when you test this with your arms?

If so, test each month of pregnancy separately and find out in which month the stress occurred.

You see, your body never forgets.

Now we come to the moment of crawling out of the womb:

Imagine your birth. Stress, yes or no?

By now you probably have quite a few questions in your head.

If you had no stress at the moment of your conception, you're one of the people on this Earth who have been truly wanted by their parents, consciously and subconsciously, which means that right at the beginning you were rewarded with the great gift of being loved simply because you're there.

All others—that is, about 90 percent of all human beings—experience the problem of not having been loved unconditionally at the beginning. So, later they try to get love in return for accomplishments, or being a good person, or helping others, or taking responsibility....

In that case, your first and most deeply rooted life program was born along with you: "I am not worth it." Welcome to the club!

If you experienced stress during your mother's pregnancy, it means that you've got another charge determining your life. Whatever the reason may have been: stress in your parents' relationship, survival fear, thoughts about an abortion, accidents, false diagnosis during preventive checkups, losses, fears of feeling overwhelmed... all events in the lives of your parents are still stored inside of you.

Nothing is forgotten which still represents a charge, and is not yet accepted with gratitude and peace.

During birth, many things can happen that are not so lovely, and for which Mother Nature had never intended. For example, when the mother is coerced into the use of oxytocics to pull the baby out faster, or being blinded with spot lights, or needing an ostomy, or not being allowed to nurse right away, or having one's eyes burned with medications.

"I will manage, I will manage totally on my own.
I will get well, I will get well
and be back on my feet.
I might need great strength for that.
But let's also not forget,
I've already managed much worse than that."

—R. Zuckowski (edited translation)

The lucky ones find a deep trust in knowing that they've mastered much worse the moment they were born. An example is when the baby's head moves through the birth channel and gets somewhat compressed in the process. This is a good thing, since the cranial bones get unsnagged like barbed hooks, and the skull can open and breathe. Babies born by cesarean need osteopathic treatments in order for the skull to breathe.

Do you want to feel the breath of your skull?

Create an atmosphere of peace and quiet around you so that you can concentrate.

Then put your hands gently at the sides of your head. Close your eyes and notice how your head is breathing very slowly: 5 to 15 times a minute. It expands to the sides, and to the front and back.

This breath is not always flowing freely, just like with pulmonary respiration. When one has a headache, the cranial breath is always blocked—one is literally "thick headed."

The cranial breath can also be "viscous" and heavy, as it is when people have asthma.

You can also test the breath of your skull: With the palms of your hands, gently press both sides of your head, and then find out if this causes stress using the arm-length test.

Gently press the front and back, and test again with your arms. In both cases, there should be no difference in arm length.

Should there be one, you can treat yourself immediately using *The Complete Healing System.*

But let's continue with your life:

There are still the kindergarten years, school experiences, puberty, first love, leaving your parents' house, education, time in the army, studying . . .

You will find strains and burdens and negative charges, no doubt. The issues we need to clear up are arranged like the layers of an onion. Each time you can only see and work on the topmost layer. Meaning that you have work to do for a few years, and it won't ever be boring.

What to do with the test results?

Very simple: You treat yourself and work with the old charges and patterns in order to discharge or release them. I deliberately don't say "delete" them; they're important experiences and only want to be integrated.

I don't program people, and I don't delete hard drives. My only goal is to be able to live now, and this requires that all old and still active charges and patterns be released from our lives, and thus resolved.

In life, we follow the old patterns and charges like well-worn paths. We walk senseless paths, go into wrong directions, choose dead-end roads—and all of this thanks to the force of habit!

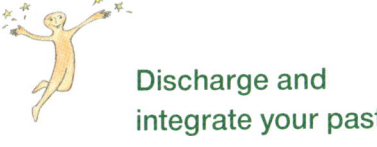

Discharge and integrate your past

Now it's time for your healing:

Think about a particular situation and treat yourself. Clear up the old charges and patterns.

Find the remedies or healing cards and work with them until you no longer react with stress. Using the copy card, you can then copy these healing cards to your *innerwise* amulet.

It's possible that your mother or your father may need a remedy as well in order to find peace.

If so, find healing cards for them, close your eyes, and imagine giving them the cards as a gift, like a bouquet of flowers. They decide if they accept the bouquet, or if they don't. If it comes from your heart without any ulterior motive, they will accept the gift. In this case, it makes no difference if they're still alive or have passed on already.

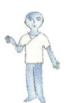 And now we come to the most wonderful application of *innerwise*: making children.

"For years we've been trying to get pregnant. We've tried everything, and you're our last hope." How often have I heard this from clients!

And now I'll show you how to make your thus far unfulfilled desire of having children a reality.

It's really very simple:

Ground rules:

1. You should test this together with your partner.
2. Then test if you're allowed to have this treatment. Without this permission you shouldn't do it.

Imagine you conceive a child.

The arm-length test will reveal that both of you feel stress in regard to this idea. This means: You both say "no."

How can something occur that both of you cannot inwardly imagine?

Now let's go into more detail.

Test the following:

1. Is it physically possible for you to conceive a child?
   Many men believe they're not worth anything if their sperm count is a few million less than average. The amount of sperm is as important for the male feeling of self-worth, as the size of his penis is, whereas one tiny sperm is enough to make a child. And many women believe that their uterus, tubes or ovaries are not good enough. So the first thing you do is get rid of these programmed feelings of inferiority. Should these feelings,

or indeed some physical condition, keep you from conceiving a child, it's often possible to solve the problem using *The Complete Healing System,* vitamins, herbs and detoxification, or test who or what can help you.

2. Now it's time for you to take a closer look at your relationship. Close your eyes and visualize how you relate to one another, as if you saw a picture before you inner eye. Are both of you equally tall in your picture? Are you standing close to each other? Do you look at each other? If both are equally tall, it means both of you carry the same amount of responsibility. Should the picture not be optimal, draw as many healing cards as allowed (using the arm-length test, ask: "Do we have permission?") until the picture is optimal. In this way, you are conducting a couple's treatment.

    It's also possible that a couple's treatment results in separation. In that case, the child would have functioned as a temporary savior of the relationship. We should not expect this kind of job from any child, but instead, look honestly at our situation and communicate with each other.

3. Now test if the two of you have a contract for common children in the first place. You can test it; or you close your eyes and visualize both of your souls and see if there's a connection from you to the soul of one or more children. Yes, you can see that. And not only that, but also how far away the child's soul still is and if perhaps there are possibly two souls who want to come together. Whenever I've seen two, these couples eventually had twins.

4. You might have a problem if only one of you has a contract with the child's soul, and the other part of the contract is with another person. Now you have to communicate very carefully, since contracts can change. When we clear up our issues, oftentimes our path in life changes, too. Life consists of forks in the road. We always have the choice as to what we want to experience. This means that after resolving an issue, there can be a contract with both of you.

5. Now visualize the moment of conception, pregnancy, the changing of the woman's body, birth, nursing, the nights of interrupted sleep (be realistic—often this lasts up to a year and a half), possibly many months without sex, and the responsibility you have for a child. If you encounter blockages, treat them.

6. If everything is fine, there are no barriers on the physical level, you stick together as a couple, have a common contract with the soul of a child; and if in the image you both see with your inner eye, this soul is already very near to you; and if you can visualize everything—from the moment of conception all the way to holding your child's hand walking through the park—you will have a big surprise coming in the next three to four weeks.

And here is some real feedback:

"The miracle of Creation—twins, our double blessing.

Dear Uwe,

When I came into your office on December 13, 2006, with the desire to finally get pregnant, I was totally discouraged, since I had tried so many different approaches, all without success. Could it really be so easy to get pregnant? You encouraged me and were a hundred percent convinced that I would have a baby. At that time I thought: What in the world makes him so sure?

After I did a pregnancy test in January, I was totally amazed: For the first time in my 35 years it was positive!

A few days later my doctor confirmed the pregnancy, and she could hardly belief the fact that I was going to have twins!

My biggest wish has come true!

Uwe and the *innerwise* system have entirely convinced me. In my eyes it's a unique system that finally does what it promises, and it's so easy to use!

With all my heart, I wish that every woman with an unfulfilled desire to have a child be introduced to this system so that her greatest wish may come true just as mine did.

Thank you so very much, dear Uwe!

Whole-heartedly,
Antje"

The point is not about more children coming into this world, but that more happy and whole children arrive who, with the beauty of their souls and their honesty, will change this world. There are already enough *Homo sapiens*. Now is the time for the *Homo integer*.

With *innerwise*, you can pave the way for having a baby yourselves and get the help you need in order to maintain the completion and beauty of your child.

You can determine which food is healthy for your child, which medications help and don't harm your child when it gets sick, and which vaccinations are meaningful and well-tolerated.

Or do you still believe that seven serious childhood diseases suddenly lead to better health? Multiple vaccinations are almost never well tolerated and harm the child.

The only solution:

Learn to test yourself, and enjoy your freedom.

22.

LET HE WHO IS WITHOUT SIN
CAST THE FIRST STONE . . .

When it comes to abuse, many people immediately think of sexual abuse. But what other forms of abuse are there?

When a single mother's or a single father's level of maturity is that of a five-year-old, and their three-year-old child then has to have the social maturity of a 22-year-old person to compensate for that, is that abuse? Yes, **responsibility abuse**.

Children who had to be all grown-up while they were a child, will want to be a child as an adult, which makes them partly unable to cope with life.

When adults use children as a battery and live off their energy, is that abuse? Yes, **energetic abuse**.

This is energy vampirism, and the child will not experience the world and life in its own abundance and beauty, and will fall ill more often.

When, after a separation, children are used to hurt the ex-partner or to blackmail him or her by not making decisions in the best interest of the child, is that abuse? Yes, **abuse of power**.

Using children for such "power games" is cruel.

When grown-ups take their bad mood out on children, is that abuse? Yes, **emotional abuse**.

Because the children can't fight back and oftentimes take on the bad energy like a sponge, turning into a trash can for the grown-ups' bad temper.

"The worst day in my life will be when my children (17 and 18 years old) move out." Is that abuse? Yes, **relationship abuse**.
When children constitute the only meaning of life for a parent.

Working with small children when it's obvious that they carry their parents' issues, without having worked with their parents first, is that abuse? Yes, **therapeutic abuse**.
Why? Because out of love for their parents, children take on their unsolved issues. But these are not the children's issues. When I work with a child treating the issues of his or her parents, the child gets better at first, and consequently, it can absorb even more issues from his or her parents and will slide even deeper into the role of acting like a grown-up.
Once a mother called me because her seven-year-old daughter had been running a fever for several days, and nothing helped. I suggested she herself should drink a peppermint tea, since the tests had shown that only the mother needed something. Half an hour after she had finished the tea, the daughter was free of fever.
This kind of approach requires the therapist to look beyond the symptoms and recognize the causes, while taking a close look at the overall system of the family. Nowadays that's the least one can demand of a therapist.

If we want to fill our own incompleteness, our emptiness, our loneliness with children, as often happens in relationships, and even more after a separation, when the children become a partner substitute, is that abuse? Yes, the **abuse of their soul**.

One day, an 18-year-old boy came to me who had been unable to go to school for years, all day sitting idle at home, watching television the whole time and sometimes playing the guitar. With the help of the arm-length test, we found out that he had lived in a state of total rigidity since he was 14. He was stuck in trauma. This generates a feeling of seeing an unreal world, as if through a fog, and not being able to do anything about it. When he was 14 years old, his parents had separated, his mother had left, and he had stayed with his father, who was the needier parent.

His father couldn't cope with the separation, because in many respects he was dependent on his wife. So he teamed up with his son against the mother, made him his ally and partner substitute. What could have been the social maturity of the father at that time? The test showed a six-year-old, while the child had taken on the role of a 32-year-old. That was too great a burden on his young shoulders and had cost him four years of his life. Four weeks after the father's and son's treatments, the boy returned to school, practiced his guitar regularly and once again had a clear outlook on life.

All forms of abuse are traumas and leave a charge behind that contributes to shaping one's life.

In addition, part of the soul always gets lost with a trauma. Some people perceive this as a kind of separation.

And both these aspects together prevent the trauma from healing.

 Come on Doc, enough with the drama! It seems nobody gets away unscathed. Sounds like that saying in the Bible: "Let he who is without sin cast the first stone."

Yes, you're right, it's not about throwing stones.

And as the therapist, it's not about deeply stirring up the suffering again until tears start flowing, thereby satisfying the therapist's ego. ("I'm such a hero . . .!")

But it's also not about enjoying the drama, as drama queens and drama kings love to do.

It's all about one simple word: THANK YOU.

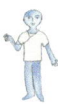 *Really Doc, now you're totally cuckoo. I'm supposed to thank the people who have hurt me?*

 You remember the chapter "Let's try saying 'thank you!'"?

I know, it's a complicated subject, therefore, here's a quick recap:

The question is: For what should we say "thank you?" The answer is: Only for what we were allowed to learn from the experience. That's all.

And with an honest and heartfelt "thank you" we can clear up and integrate the charges and become free again. The more we clear up these old energetic charges, the more we're able to really live in the present.

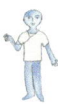 *Oh boy! Dear reader, I got a hunch what drill is coming next. Maybe you better stop reading immediately and return to the bookstore where you bought it and try to get your money back. Or even better, give it to all those people who may thank you for an experience in life—in the hope they survive this part of it.*

But honestly Doc, does it really work?

 If you just write on your mirror "thank you" 100 times, probably not. Doing so only allows the part of the iceberg that lies above the water to write, and you remember the block of shares.

The entire iceberg has to say THANK YOU. This is best done if you imagine standing before this person, looking him or her in the eyes and into the heart and saying: "Thank you for this experience. It wasn't easy, but I know that my soul had a part in planning it. It has made me richer, richer in experience."

When was the last time you surprised yourself with a bouquet of flowers? Celebrate and enjoy yourself.

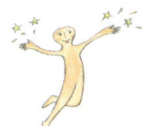

Saying "thank you"

And here's more inspiration for the brave:

Say "thank you" to three people who have gifted you with an important experience in your life. You can call them, send them an e-mail or a classic handwritten letter or say it directly to their face.

If you cannot reach this person for any reason, imagine that you are both facing each other, and are able to look into each other's eyes and hearts.

And then say to one another: "Thank you for making this experience possible for me."

And don't forget to thank the people to whom you owe positive experiences.

There is the story about two angels who meet in heaven and tell each other what they've learned in their lives as humans.

One of them says: "I've experienced all there is, but there is one thing I haven't learned: how to forgive."

The second angel says: "Next time I can help you experience it, if you like."

"You would do that for me? You are a true friend, and I love you," says the other angel in response.

The second angel looks deep into the eyes of his friend and says: "Please never forget that you have asked me do to this."

23.

THE BIG CLEAN-UP:
FIRST YOUR HOME, THEN YOUR LIFE

*How much are you willing to change
if you are not doing well?
If your conditions are a result of the way you
lead your life, it's only logical to change your life
so your conditions can improve.*

A woman I know called me and asked for a treatment. She complained that she couldn't be happy anymore. I refused the treatment. I only asked her to sense if there was any sadness when visualizing being alone on an island. She said: "No, because then I am free again."

So the medicine I gave her was the advice to go away for a few days, alone, without her partner, and to take more time for herself in the future. Then her partner would also have a chance for development. To this she said: "I was afraid you would say that."

I simply don't want to dispense pills for happiness anymore. I've also changed my life time and again, even radically, when necessary.

Mr. Mind, please say once:

"I am ready to change everything in order to live a healthy and happy life again!"

That's something I have to think through first. Everything? Do you really mean everything?

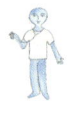 Oh well, it depends how much you still want to suffer. Change everything in your life that pulls down your energy. All compromises, for example.

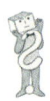 *How much time do I have for that?*

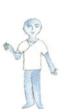 All the time in the world. After all, it's *your* life!

I know some patients with cancer who went to the Philippines to get help from spiritual surgeons.

Here they needed a wheelchair, had no more strength and didn't want to eat anymore. There, they got daily treatments that removed the cancer from their body. They prayed, went for walks on the beach and were able to eat again. They were feeling fine.

When the two or three weeks of treatment were over, and they were on their way back home, some of them collapsed as soon as they were on the plane, and six months later half of those patients had died from cancer, despite the fact that they were free of it during their time in the Philippines.

I'm sure that after a few months in the Philippines, they would have started to continue their old way of life and developed the illness once again, paradise or not.

We can't run away from ourselves.

Sure, we can escape for a while, but our shadow always catches up with us. Or we can end our old relationships, and after some time with a new partner, we find ourselves stuck in the same old patterns.

I once met a couple in Australia who left everything behind in order to save their relationship. Since the man had had an affair, they moved to a place more than 1,000 miles away in order to start anew.

If they are lucky, this action will give them a respite of one year or so. Then, their shadow will catch up with them, and everything will be as it was before.

So, what is time Mr. Mind?

I am much more interested in how much courage you have to really change EVERYTHING!

I know you're a bit overwhelmed right now. Therefore, don't start the changes in your *own* life.

Work on other things first, as usual.

And who is least capable to fight back? Right, your house or your apartment, and the memories conserved there.

Can you breathe freely in your home? Do you feel as free there as you do near the beach or on a mountain?

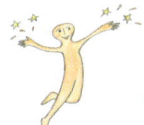

Time for housecleaning

You probably have many things in your house, your apartment, your room that you don't need anymore. Throw all of it away.

The old love letters from ex-boyfriends or ex-girlfriends that you keep in case you feel lonely again. The heirlooms full of stories that aren't yours, and which you would never have chosen for your home. Regardless of whether it's a sideboard from great-granny, or the favorite coffee cup of some aunt. The cheap, yet useless, bargain buys. Get rid of them! Books you haven't read in years, and won't read again. Pictures from the past reminding you again and again of your mortality. And the useless food processor that you have bought for the fifteenth time. Open every cabinet, every wardrobe, and free them from all the useless stuff. And don't forget the secondary rooms: the shed, garage, basement and attic. Are there still some boxes from your last move 25 years ago, with very important things you absolutely need? Simply dispose of everything that you don't really love, that is not beautiful, and not urgently needed. Away it goes into the trash, to the secondhand shop, the clear out table—it can go anywhere as long as it's gone for good! Yes, it was clutter that robbed you of your freedom and choked your breath.

I know the job is too big to be done in one day. Take your calendar, and starting today, mark as many days for the job as you may need. One room each day is a good solution. My advice: Don't allow yourself any serious breaks. Finish it.

 This gave you time to get some practice, and now the moment has come to clean up your life.

 Why? After all, my life is rather good as it is.

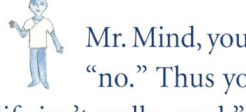 Mr. Mind, you yourself say "rather." This word is a small "no." Thus your statement reads as follows: "Well, my life isn't really good."

You coward; as a brain you simply have no spine but only spinal marrow. And that can bend easily.

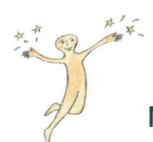

My life as a blueprint for a garden

This chart is going to be as effective as a trip to the spiritual surgeons in the Philippines, but will last longer.

Take a large piece of paper, or the free page in this book, and intuitively draw your life as a mind map. Don't think about how it should look, instead follow your feeling while you draw.

It's very easy: Imagine you draw a blueprint for a garden, with you being the garden. Now draw the following: your family, your house, your past, your job, your friends, your foes, your lovers, your lies, your creativity, your joy, your happiness . . . everything that constitutes your life. One thing you draw here, the other one there; one is smaller, the other bigger; one is squashed into a corner, the other one has a lot of space. Exactly as you would sketch in plants, trees, paths and ponds.

Has the garden turned out beautiful? Or do you have to re-plant something, clear, cut back or plant new? Is your garden overgrown with weeds? Does it get enough light? Is something missing in your garden? Do the branches of the neighbor's trees extend too much into your garden?

Now you have to make a basic decision: Do you enjoy being in your garden? Is it really your garden, or are all those plants and trees well meant gifts and advice from other people? Did you ever want your garden to be like it is now? Can you beautify it, or is it time to move on and plant a new garden somewhere else?

Of course, you are the architect of your life. Sure, like Mr. Mind you, too, can make excuses by saying it was your subconscious, in case you want to continue playing the role of the victim.

I personally maintain that our lives are an insider job, everything homemade. All happiness, all suffering, all joy, all illness, all success and all loss—everything self-made.

I am ready to change **EVERYTHING** in order to live a healthy and happy life again.

Small hint for the reader: The operative word here is **EVERYTHING**.

24.

YES TO LOVE!

"At the Paralympic Games some time ago, nine athletes—all of them mentally or physically challenged—were standing at the starting line for the 100-meter race.

Then came the starting shot, and the race began. One young man stumbled, fell down and started to cry.

The others heard the crying.

They slowed down and turned around to see what was happening.

They went back to the starting line. All eight of them. One girl with Down syndrome sat down beside the crying boy, embraced him and asked: 'You feel better now?'

Then all nine crossed the finish line together, shoulder to shoulder."

—Unknown author

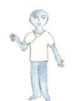 *Will you come up with another statement now, like the one about changing everything? Just a few more pages, and then I'm done with this.*

Yes, I will:
I love myself as I was, as I am and as I will be!

You can't be serious!
I shall love myself for everything I've ever done? Even though I've made mistakes, have been guilty, have failed and have been a complete a—hole?!?

And when I look at my life right now, it's obvious that half of it is simply not true.

I can't love myself for the fact that every day, I'm working in a job that I hate, but that pays me well; that I've been wanting to leave my partner, but have to wait until the kids are on their own.

I'm supposed to love me for all the lies in my life? Never ever!!

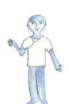
Here is another one:
I love and am loved.
I can see the lovable core in every human being and let every human being see the lovable core in me.

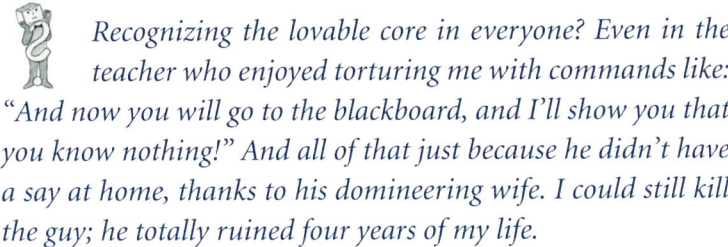

Recognizing the lovable core in everyone? Even in the teacher who enjoyed torturing me with commands like: "And now you will go to the blackboard, and I'll show you that you know nothing!" And all of that just because he didn't have a say at home, thanks to his domineering wife. I could still kill the guy; he totally ruined four years of my life.

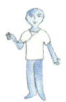
Oh my, did I ever stir up a hornet's nest here!
So let's clarify this:

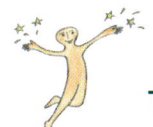

The "non-lovable" list

A. Facts from my past for which I can't love myself:

1. _____
2. _____
3. _____

B. Why I can't love myself now:

1. _____
2. _____
3. _____

C. Why I won't love myself in the future:

1. _____
2. _____
3. _____

And since you're at it, please write down the names of five people in your life whose lovable core you can't or don't want to see:

1. _____
2. _____
3. _____
4. _____
5. _____

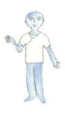 For many years, we've been offering a great exercise in our workshops. Here it is:

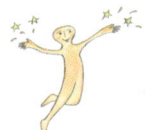
The house-sharing community

Take the list of the five people whose lovable core you can't see, and imagine living together with them in the same household. If you want, you can also choose a small island, and only you and these people are living there.

Now imagine each of these five people as your roommate or co-islander. That will surely cause stress when you do the arm-length test. Now take *The Complete Healing System* from *innerwise* and draw cards to balance the stress. Then read the description on the cards and find the issue. Now you know your issue and can work with it, since human beings are mirrors for each other. When another person triggers something in you, he or she is in resonance with your issue. These people help us by showing us our weak points.

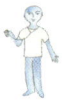 There is a saying: "Love yourself, and it doesn't matter who you marry."

And since you've already begun treating yourself, you may start to balance each and every point on your "non-lovable" list.

I love myself as I was, as I am and as I will be.

Dear Mr. Mind, you said:

"I shall love myself for everything I ever did? Even though I've made mistakes, have been guilty, have failed and have been a complete a—hole?!?"

Yes, you shall. Love yourself for everything you ever did, are doing now, and are going to do in the future.

There are no mistakes in life. It only becomes a mistake when we look back at something and realize that we would not do it in the same way now. However, we completely forget that, thanks to these experiences, we have become what we are now. Only through what we now call a "mistake" were we able to gain this insight.

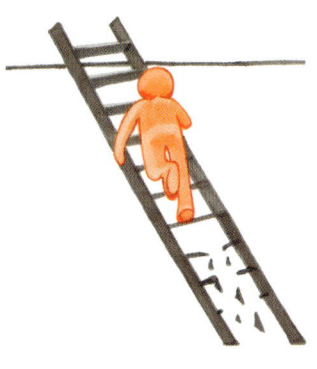

You can compare this with climbing a ladder, while you say to each step you took: "Your are a mistake, never again shall I put my foot on you. It was already a mistake to have done it in the first place."

From the viewpoint of a grown-up, it may also be a mistake to wet your bed (or something worse). When you're just starting to learn to talk, or are still in diapers, and you proudly say to your parents: "Made poo poo," they will laugh with delight and think you're unbelievably sweet.

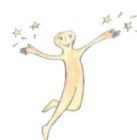

Looking others in the eyes

Look into the eyes of the people you meet; allow them to see your innermost being, your core. It's fun to do this in the open and to observe how differently people react.

The following lines are my children's gift on the occasion of my 44th birthday:

Thank you, Dad

Thank you for showing us that it doesn't matter what others think about us, as long as we're happy.

Thank you for giving us freedom by being a living example for us.

Thank you for letting us feel what true love means!
We love you! We believe that true love means to love someone *because* he or she *is*, not for what he or she is.

Thank you for always being there for us, regardless of where you are or how far away you are.

Thank you for showing us what honesty really means.

Thank you for showing us that nothing is impossible, if we really want it.

Thank you for having *sooo* much confidence in us.

Thank you for simply being the way you are, and for letting us be the way we are.

Thank you for helping us find our own path, whatever it may be.

**I love myself as I was,
as I am and as I will be.**

25.

YES TO THE BODY!

 And now I have a wonderful parameter for you: the biological age.

This helps you determine how old your body is and how fresh your cells are.

There are children whose biological age is older than 70, and 90-year-olds with a biological age of 18 years.

It has nothing to do with their chronological age.

After an octuple vaccination even a child can look seriously old.

The ideal would be if the biological age of grown-ups is at least 20 years younger than their chronological age.

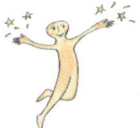 **Test your biological age in years**

Today my biological age is: _____ years.

 Now I'll show you how to do your own body check, without taking a blood sample or x-rays, and with no waiting time in doctors' offices.

How is the state of your organs, fluids, nervous system and teeth? Do you have infections, allergies or deficiencies? How is your stance, your breath and your balance?

Before we start the body check, remember that we consist of several levels. The:

- structural level (such as cells, organs)
- biochemical level (metabolism, hormones)
- mental level (thoughts)
- emotional level (feelings)
- energetic level (meridians, chakras, aura)
- spiritual level (soul, soul plan)

Now it might be a good idea if you go on the Internet and do a crash course in anatomy so you know where the organs are located.

If your heart hurts, there might be a problem on the organic level, or it might be emotionally broken. In any case, it hurts.

And now let's start with the body diagnostics:

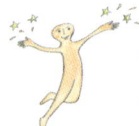

Video clip 14 Testing your organs
Testing your organs

With the arm-length test you can find imbalances.

If, for example, you lightly press your belly in the area where you liver is located, and afterward testing shows a difference in arm length, it means that your liver is stressed. No more and no less. To find out which level of your liver feels the stress, you can say and test the following words:

- Liver on the structural level
- Liver on the biochemical level
- Liver on the mental level
- Liver on the emotional level
- Liver on the spiritual level

In this way, the arm-length test reveals the affected levels.

The liver is the organ where anger, rage, resentment and swallowed feelings are stored. We all know expressions such as: not wanting to look at something; being heartbroken; crying one's eyes out, coughing one's lungs out, something makes one's blood boil, etc.

Our illnesses almost always begin as irritations on the spiritual, energetic and emotional levels.

It's only a question of time until an irritation—for instance, on the energetic and emotional levels—manifests itself also on the physical level and then reflects in changed laboratory results. And ultimately—years later—ultrasounds and x-rays show an alteration.

The dentist only sees a change in the bone underneath a tooth when half of the bone is already corroded. That's pretty late because the infection has been poisoning the body for years. But your tooth started hurting long before that.

Here's an overview of important organs so you can mark them right away and also note the appropriate remedy that you test in case an organ is problematic.

If you can't restore balance in an organ, you should see your doctor or therapist.

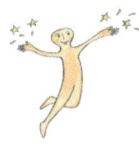 **Video clip 15 Testing your breathing**

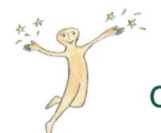 **Organ check**

Organ tested	Balance	Stress	Balancing healing cards or remedies
Liver			
Gallbladder			
Stomach			
Pancreas			
Spleen			
Blood			
Lymph			
Adrenal glands			
Kidneys			
Urethra, bladder			
Small intestine			
Large intestine			
Testicles, prostate,			
Vagina, uterus			
Fallopian tubes, ovaries			
Parasympathetic nervous system: pelvic plexus, cranial nerves			
Sympathetic nervous system: cervical plexus, solar plexus			
Diaphragm			
Breasts			
Heart			
Lungs			
Thyroid			
Teeth			
Sinuses			
Tonsils			
Ears			
Eyes			
Brain			
Nerves			
Skin			

If you test your organs regularly, say once a week or once a month, by touching your body where the respective organs are located and concentrating on it, you can detect any irritation very early and still correct it with simple remedies.

Even with already existing symptoms, you can still touch the painful areas. They will generate a difference in arm length, and then you can find the appropriate remedy—water, herbs, vitamins, colors . . . or healing cards—until you can again touch the organ or think about the symptom without getting a difference in arm length.

If everybody does that, soon our health insurance contributions will drop below five percent!

Here are some more tips from experience:

If you have a *lumbago*, kidney tea often works miracles because these irritations are based on tension in the segment-indicating muscles of the kidneys, the so-called iliopsoas muscles.

Rashes and *eczema* can often be treated successfully with liver or gallbladder teas.

Attention: Supplements with *algae*, such as Chlorella, should always be taken in combination with kidney tea containing goldenrod; otherwise the kidneys will become overwhelmed by the amount of toxins released.

After checking the organs, we will now take a closer look at your diet: Are you well nourished?

- What nourishes your heart, your brain, your desire for touch, your cells and your soul?
- We nourish ourselves with everything we eat, see, feel, drink, hear, dream, think and touch.
- Do you nourish your brain with positive or negative thoughts?

- Do you nourish your heart with envy, jealousy, greed, etc. or with love, generosity and openness?
- Do you surround yourself with light or dark energies?
- Do you nourish your soul by living your life purpose?
- What do you eat? What do you drink?

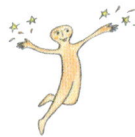

Testing your nutritional status

I am nourished on all levels:	Yes	No	I am missing
emotional			
energetic			
spirituel			
mental			
physical			

 Did you ever think about what was or is the greatest poison in your life?

Well, the first things that come to mind are amalgam and wood preservatives. But wait, there was something else: my ex-wife. And if I think about it even harder, I always felt that my parents didn't really love me. That was even worse.

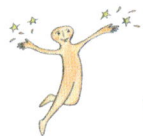

Your poison check

My poisons are:	Yes	No	Detoxification with:
thoughts			
emotions			

My poisons are:	Yes	No	Detoxification with:
energies			
memories			
chemicals			
metals			
life situations			
other			

Now you have to be careful when testing. You ask: "Am I poisoned?" If you are, your body responds with "yes," your arms are equally long.

Since your body can only say "yes" or "no," you have to pay attention to the meaning of the answer to your question. Having equally long arms is not always a positive thing.

Should you have gotten "yes" as an answer, right away you test the appropriate remedies for detoxification.

More than 80 percent of our body consists of water, and when we are thirsty, it's always a thirst for water.

Neither coffee nor tea can quench thirst. They only burden the body with additional harmful substances. If your body smells bad at times, it's almost always because it's excreting the pollutants from coffee, black or green tea, or chocolate. So, if you like to quit using deodorant in the future, drink more water!

Of course, I mean still, non-carbonated water.

Depending on where you live, tap water can be a good alternative.

Even the old ritual of blessing the food had its purpose. We can substantially improve the energy of our food by blessing it with our hands. Try it with wine or water—both even taste different afterward.

26.

Finally happy!

What is happiness anyway? Where does happiness come from? Why does it always slip through our fingers like sand? Is it possible to be permanently happy? And would people be happier if they were permanently happy, or do we need ups and downs? What about the interplay of light and shadow? What is *flow*?

What do you mean with "flow?"

Imagine you're a pipe. You can be very narrow and calcified, and not much can flow through you anymore. Or you can be wide and open; then a lot of light will flow through you. And you can be so wide open that you don't even sense the limits of the pipe, which means you're in an extreme state of flow.

I've experienced flow in several gradations:

1. **Basic flow** is the basic trust in life that you don't have to struggle any longer. You're taken care of, everything arrives at the right time, and you have long ago ceased to believe in coincidences. To experience flow, your own identity has to be clear: I am I = yes. You only have your own energy field and are not carrying the burden for ten other people. And you've found peace. The big traumas in your life are healed, and you have retrieved the lost fragments of your soul.

Reaching this state already requires quite a bit of work, and—as described before—you can do it yourself. It involves the daily effort to maintain this state of being, and it's well worth it. Once you're accustomed to the basic flow, the "normal" blocked state will no longer be a livable alternative for you.

2. In the state of **extreme flow** you begin to shine. You feel a tingling all over, and an infinite stream of creative power and joy flows through you. You feel one with everything. Your freedom knows no bounds, and you feel light. Your body dances.

**Happiness is
the expression of flow pervading us**

- In a state of narrowness we are like a thin pipe with very little light flowing through it.
- In a state of expansiveness we are like a wide pipe with lots of light flowing through it.
- In a state of openness we *are* the flow of light.

The light flowing through us makes us happy and creative.

- In a state of narrowness the room around the pipe of light is filled with a lot of darkness.
- In a state of expansiveness part of this darkness is already transformed.
- In a state of openness the room is filled with light, and there is no more room for darkness.

Darkness feeds the sadness, fear and envy in us.

Recognizing the darkness in us, and transforming it through healing work, gives us the strength to change from a thin pipe of light to a wide pipe of light, and ultimately to become the flow of light ourselves.

Then we are finally happy. The pipe is our *I*, our Self, and what I call the *ego*.

Wait a minute, Doc! Now I got to ask you something.
What happens if I don't have my own identity? The ego *is a no-no among new-agers; it is something that must be obliterated. One Kundalini practice is even called the "ego eraser." But listening to you, it sounds as if the* ego *is not that bad after all?*

 Our own identity is an absolute requirement for us to live a happy life.

80 percent of my clients have lost it. When they come to see me and do the arm-length test, the answer to "I am I" is always "no."

Then I always ask: "Who are you if you're not you?" Big baffled eyes.

My next question is: "And whose life is it you're living?"

And then the room gets very quiet.

If you don't have your identity:

- Things happen that make you feel you don't need this experience, such as accidents und injuries.
- You struggle but don't seem to get any closer to your goals.
- You want to live authentically, but it doesn't work.
- You take on illnesses and burdens that aren't yours.
- You even have pain that isn't yours.
- You feel energetically empty.

Now imagine decision-makers like a chancellor or a president, have lost their own identity. All those campaign promises are not true anymore. Who is governing then?

Or closer to the action in your personal life: Your children come back from a visit with grandma, or a play date, and somehow they're different. After one or two hours they're finally back with you, body and soul, and you can feel them. They needed this time to find their own identity again.

And, let's not forget the old ego issue.

Even as an adult, I tried to heal, cleanse and remove my ego; to be ego-less, and to live devoted to what is good.

One whole year I struggled and fought with my ego. I underwent emotional therapy, conquered the pain during yoga, felt miserable as soon as the "bad" ego reared its ugly head again, and let my partner tell me how desperately necessary it was for me to free myself from the ego. It was an interesting journey through the therapeutic netherworld.

When the only success my self-therapy showed was that my feeling of self-worth hit rock bottom, I understood that after all, the ego issue was not my problem. Instead, I had tried to see the selfishness and egotism of my partner as my problem, and in the process had simply lost myself.

I love my ego. *Ego* means *I*. And I can give a lot of love to this *I*. All creative power comes through this *I*. It's the space which makes it possible to be happy and creative.

I have a few more questions: What's the deal with "dark energy?" Why do some people have such dark energy that one feels disgusted and doesn't want to be physically close to them? Wouldn't it be better to live in a temple in Tibet where there are only light human beings?

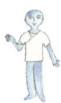 Maybe that's possible in a remote temple in Tibet. I haven't visited one yet.

However, I want to live here, have a rather normal life with children and friends, go out dancing and have fun, and remain fit to live my daily life here. If I only lived in an artificial environment as a "light" human being, I would be a prisoner of my spiritual search. Bye-bye freedom!

I've experienced some spiritual communities in the Western world. I wouldn't want to live in most of those. These are not places of enlightenment, but just extremely well functioning places to supply the respective guru with energy. Some of those places remind me of cowsheds where the animals are regularly milked, a price they willingly pay so they don't feel lost and lonely anymore.

Sects show similar structures, though oftentimes they have more sophisticated systems to make people dependent on them so that they can take their most valuable treasure: their heart energy.

There it is again, the old fable of the cold heart—still applicable today.

Light and shadow—the prevailing issue that none of us can bypass.

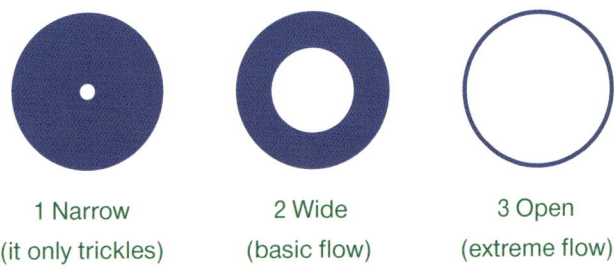

Light and darkness comprise one system.

1. If the light is narrow, darkness fills the space.
2a. The expansion of light transforms darkness. Most energetic light workers concentrating only on the positive would agree with that.
2b. Viewed differently: With the transformation of darkness, light expands. Process workers who try to work through the traumas of the past until they're cleared up would agree with this.
3. Once the space is filled with light, there is no more room for darkness.

Some people describe this path the other way around. They transform the light into darkness, gaining power in return. This is the great temptation for broken souls.

Since actively facing the dark side creates our impetus to understand life and to search for the light, we're not spared from coming into daily contact with darkness, as long as we resonate with it.

And we can always choose to not let dark, energy-sucking people back into our lives, even if they're our friends, parents or present partners. Though the fact is, we can't entirely avoid the dark side itself. If necessary, it would catch up with us even in a monastery in Tibet.

If you want to know how far you've already come on your way to the Light, you can test the following:

How much of your creative potential do you live?

You can measure it in percentages.

My actual creative potential expressed in life is _____%.

Though remember to look at yourself from outside using spherical vision so you don't deceive yourself.

Here, an empirical value as a reference: Results from one to five percent are normal. In this case you simply know you still got a long bucket list.

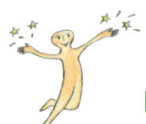

Bucket list

What else would you like to experience before you kick the bucket?

The wonderful movie *The Bucket List* with Morgan Freeman and Jack Nicholson is about two men with cancer living out their bucket list. Life gives them the necessary time to do this.

What is on your bucket list?

And how long will you wait until you finally live it out?

What I want to experience before I kick the bucket:

- _____
- _____
- _____
- _____
- _____
- _____
- _____
- _____

Tell me Doc, what does being happy mean to you?

Being able to breathe freely.
Your face glows.
You dance through life.
Your body is light.
You live in the present.
Your happiness is highly contagious.
Your life has a purpose.
You're full of creative power.
You vibrate with energy.
Your body consists solely of rhythms.
Your heart is wonderfully warm and strong.
You're open; you don't need protection anymore.
Your struggles are over, you are given everything you need.
You're thankful for everything that you've experienced so far.
It's wonderful to be a human being.
Nature is made of colors, shapes and sounds;
you've never felt like this before.
You're not alone anymore since everything around you
is starting to come alive.
You have many creative ideas, and the strength and
courage to live them out.

In case anyone here is still interested in my opinion, I can only say this to you: Happiness comes from me, the heart. A happy heart attracts more happiness. That is called resonance. As Connor Mayfield used to say: "Happiness comes to the happy."

27.

WHEN YOU'RE IN THE FLOW, SUCCESS IS INEVITABLE

 The moment of truth regarding your inner programs for success is near.

First we will address the fear factor.

When it comes to success, the number one big preventer is fear. Number two is also fear, and the same goes for number three.

There are only two basic driving forces in our lives: fear and trust.

Presently, the global field of consciousness is determined by fear by a rate of more than 80 percent, and the situation is hardly different when it comes to the individual.

On average, between 60 to 95 percent of people's main driving force is fear. This doesn't mean however that fear is visible on the surface, but it's the deepest driving force.

With *unsuccessful* people, the fear factor is over 85 percent, while *successful* people have a fear factor that is under 65 percent.

I've also seen people with more than 95 percent fear: one failure after the other, plus several lawsuits and litigations simultaneously.

Creative force can only manifest itself through us if we're confident. Control and manipulation are the results of fear. If we want to do without these two crooks, we have to transform fear into confidence and trust.

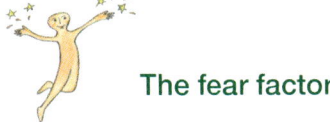
The fear factor

My fear factor in %: _____

This remedy helps me outgrow fear:
_____
_____

This activity helps me outgrow fear:
_____
_____

Now I'll show you how to work with projects, systems and companies. In my opinion, these are also living systems. This means they're subject to the same laws, and are to be treated with the same method.

How do I talk to a company? Whose arms shall I take, the janitor's or the boss's?

Just your own. You can test with your hands by proxy, if you don't forget to use spherical vision.

*Okay, I'm an employee in a company and want a pay raise. So I go to an **innerwise** coach and let him do some of his magic, and—voilà! I get more money.*

You don't seem to know the unwritten laws of therapists. Any therapist or coach who tries to do this kind of trickery gets a real punch on the nose from the universe. I've seen therapists who, after such an incident, were unable to do energy work for many months because they had misused their powers.

Ground rule no. 1:
You always need permission. In this case, only the person responsible for the pay raise can give it. You're only allowed to work from the top down, never the other way around.

Ground rule no. 2:
Always look at the issue objectively. Always work for the highest good of everyone involved.

Ground rule no. 3:
You may dissolve energies or send them back to the addresser, but never add anything. The goal is to always allow the person sending the energetic manipulations to learn something. It should never be about revenge.

If you want to work on your project or your company, you need to start with an overview.

Take some different-colored pencils or pens and a big piece of paper. And now get started: Draw your company, your project . . .

Draw how you feel it emotionally. It's quite possible that you find the cleaning lady in the center, or the secretary. Though these two surely don't belong there.

In regard to a certain company, for example, the drawing revealed that an employee stood in the middle, dominating everything else. The bosses didn't have much say. The moment when everybody could see the position of power she had earned thanks to her erotic dallying with the boss, the employee got really angry. With one drawing, ten years of hard, subversive, sweat-inducing work to gain power turned into a total waste of time.

Ideally, the core of the project, or what a company is really working for, needs to be in the center.

With a school, it's the children. With a business, it can be the product or the basic values; with a research project, it would be the discovery or the invention. I would never put the money in the center, since the goal should never be money; rather, money should be available in the necessary abundance because it is a good project.

Write your wishes and goals down for your project or business. Then imagine they have come true, and test it. It can be a sobering experience if success generates stress for you.

How can something occur if not even the subconscious of the boss believes in it?

Using your intuition, add all the important elements to the drawing and then test if all deciding factors, people, etc. are there. Continue until everything and everybody is present in your drawing.

Now test if the place that the individual elements occupy is optimal for them. Then test if the relationship between those elements is stress-free.

Now you work with the drawing as you would with a human being: You place healing cards on the elements that need something until all stress is gone, leaving the cards on the drawing.

Next, you draw all of this again on a new piece of paper. You'll be amazed by how much the picture has already changed.

Then you look at the constellation again and test the positions and interactions. If necessary, continue working with the elements that need treatment, and draw again.

Oftentimes, three drawings are all you need to reach your goal: **flow in the entire system**. All blockages are removed, each element has found its optimal position and the system is open to evolve again.

Now you can test how long the drawings and their healing cards have to remain untouched. This could be months. Or you store the healing symphony on the *innerwise* discs for system treatments so the healing cards are not blocked any longer.

Next you test your goals and wishes again. A miracle has happened. . . .

> Reality follows energy. You've designed an ideal energy field; you've created a hologram of the optimum. Now reality will very soon adjust to this frame of reference and develop accordingly. You'll be amazed how fast this can be when you've considered all factors.

For systems and companies or organizations, it makes sense to have an independent person test the result again.

It's simply exhilarating to see projects in the flow. Everything happens by itself. We only have to accept it.

This was a short overview to make your mouth water. You can now begin with your projects using spherical vision. Working with projects and businesses is more complex than working with individuals, since you need to consider so many aspects simultaneously and have to stay on top of things. Even if you forget just one aspect, it will affect the entire situation.

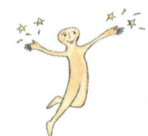

Your success check

	Yes	No	Remedies, healing cards
I am happy.			
My profession is my calling.			
I earn enough money.			
I enjoy my success.			
I am honest with myself.			
I am honest with others.			
I like to take responsibility for tasks.			
I love my work.			
I deserve to be successful.			
I am good.			
I accomplish my tasks with a high degree of quality.			
I am competent in my area. I like to make decisions.			
I enjoy taking responsibility.			
I am open to new things.			
I am open to changes.			

28.

THE GREAT MOTHER

 Most people I know have mother issues.
But is it really about the biological mother? Are there really that many unfit mothers?

I think it's about something completely different, and the biological mother serves as a projection screen.

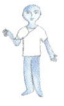 *You just about saved your neck among our female readers.*

 Can you imagine that the Earth is a living being?
Really alive and breathing, with a heart, a soul, rhythms, cycles, pimples and scars?

Ancient cultures called her the Great Mother.

She is alive, she has a soul, she can love, erupt and tremble.

She has veins with water and oil flowing through them.

And we are her pimples. Little bumps who, from her perspective, disappear rather quickly. If you have a problem with thinking of yourself as a pimple, you may call yourself a bud. However, it doesn't change the fast ticking away of time.

Everything our body consists of comes from her, and she lives through us.

This means that we are children of the Great Mother.

And not only us; everything that exists is made of Mother Earth.

This includes every computer, every tree, every banana, every plastic bag and every chemical factory . . . simply everything that exists on Earth. Nothing was delivered here via spaceship.

Hey, by now you might start to feel some resistance: After all, chemical factories are not in the slightest biodynamic enterprises. And a plastic bag is a bad thing.

In the eyes of the Earth, what are one million years until all these things we have burdened her with have decomposed? We just think in terms of extremely short cycles and call it "environmental pollution." Mother Earth can keep on living despite a short-lived rash. Time will heal it. But for us it *is* a problem, since we only have 100 years to live.

The wax in your ears, your fragrant excretions and jealous thoughts are also part of you, are they not? Or do you really want to tell me you're only your loving heart, your humbleness and goodness; that you're a pure angel beyond any duality?

95 percent of our universe consists of dark matter. We can't even see it, and yet it exists and pervades everything. And in our limitless arrogance as little humans, we deem ourselves able to define laws of nature, to give students grades for the present state of general ignorance and to declare what is good and what is bad—all based on the fraction of the five percent of matter that we *do* understand.

Humanity as a whole doesn't behave differently from Mr. Mind with his one to five percent of the shares. A know-it-all, but for the most part insignificant.

Before we arrive at the reunion with the Great Mother, here are some practical pre-tests so you can comprehend what this may mean for your life:

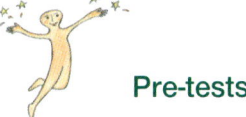

Pre-tests

1. Get yourself into a relaxed position and imagine you are standing on a balancing beam. Now you lift up your arms and do a cartwheel on the balancing beam. So, how was it? Did you land safely? Or did you stumble and are now lying on the floor? Or did you just wobble a bit?

My cartwheel on the balancing beam was:

_____

2. Now let's look at your choppers—at least at those still in their original state. Maybe you think they're fixed, immovable? Wrong. Normally, each tooth can move freely: to the front, to the back, and with very light turns—you may say they can dance. That's their normal state. Though in most people that isn't the case. Their teeth are either too fixed, or they're pulled and shoved in different directions, and the idea of free movement generates stress; like patronized and controlled children, they're not free anymore.

Teeth			Teeth		
First quadrant (upper right)		Second quadrant (upper left)	First quadrant (upper right)		Second quadrant (upper left)
18 17 16 15 14 13 12 11		21 22 23 24 25 26 27 28	1 2 3 4 5 6 7 8		9 10 11 12 13 14 15 16
48 47 46 45 44 43 42 41		31 32 33 34 35 36 37 38	32 31 30 29 28 27 26 25		24 23 22 21 20 19 18 17
Fourth quadrant (lower right)		Third quadrant (lower left)	Fourth quadrant (lower right)		Third quadrant (lower left)
Europe			Amerika		

Now you can control this with the arm-length test. Move your teeth back and forth with your tongue and imagine them turning slightly. Simultaneously test with your arms if this generates stress.

Repeat this with every tooth in your upper and lower jaw.

3. Your brain waves are the voice of your brain, and according to their function, we discern them as follows:

- Delta waves: 1 to 4 hertz, typical for the dreamless phase of deep sleep
- Theta waves: 4 to 8 hertz, typical for light phases of sleep
- Alpha waves: 8 to 13 hertz, typical for deep relaxation
- Beta waves: 13 to 30 hertz, typical for the waking state
- Gamma waves: more than 30 hertz, typical for intense concentration and learning processes

Next test whether your brain is able to communicate perfectly in all frequency ranges.

Brain communication works perfectly in the area of:

Delta waves	◯ Yes	◯ No
Theta waves	◯ Yes	◯ No
Alpha waves	◯ Yes	◯ No
Beta waves	◯ Yes	◯ No
Gamma waves	◯ Yes	◯ No

Maybe through meditation you're familiar with the idea of letting roots grow into the earth in order to ground yourself. As for me, I always found the idea of roots a bit funny. Are you an alien who finds him- or herself on a strange planet digging his roots into the ground to siphon something off or hang on to something?

No, you're a child of the Great Mother Earth, possibly separated from her, but you have never been anything other than a part of her. Forget the idea of the roots. After all, you're a bud of the Great Mother.

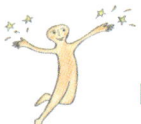

Mom, I'm coming home

Take some time for this exercise.
  Sit or lay down relaxed.
  Begin to notice again the rhythms of the Great Mother, feel her heart, her warmth and her love, and again become one with her.

Now say:

> "Mother Earth,
> as a part of you,
> you are fully in me
> and live through me."

If this statement generates stress when you feel it, say it or do the arm-length test, balance the stress: with colors, crystals, flowers or the healing cards.

 This is the connection to the Great Mother—now on to the father: our Sun.

The root of all religions is Sun worship. Those three days of Jesus on the cross are a synonym for the winter solstice at the Southern Cross. The devil is the night. The resurrection is the moment when the day again begins to be longer than the night. For this reason, the life-giving Sun was equated with the Divine.

It represents the fatherly aspect, like the *yang* in Chinese philosophy: activity, growth, heat, conception and day.

At this point a small digression to the war of the sexes, if I may:

It constitutes a profound misinterpretation to think that women have been oppressed in the last few thousand years. These are victim games that don't bring healing to anyone; they only generate more pain and war. We find an unbelievable amount of hardened and bitter people, especially among feminists.

Neither women nor men were being oppressed, but the masculine and feminine aspects in every human being.

Thus, it would make sense if men created a "femininity movement" to once again feel and live out their own female side.

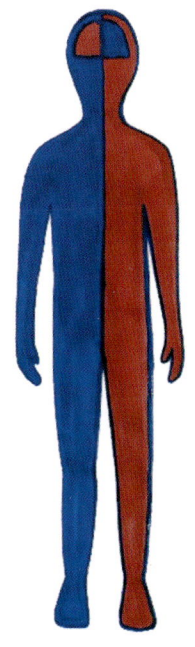

Our left cerebral hemisphere and the right side of our body symbolize male energy, while the right hemisphere and the left side of the body represent female energy.

Why do some people repeatedly have symptoms on only *one* side of the body?

What does it mean when the left leg is shorter, or when the right side of the chest doesn't open up properly when inhaling?

And why are only people with a dominant left-brain hemisphere able to cope with a PC, whereas all others go nuts when trying to work with it? Though as soon as they get their hands on an Apple computer, they're ecstatic and will never again voluntarily change to a PC.

Another misinterpretation is the assumption that men can do only one thing at a time, whereas women can do many things simultaneously. The masculine side in us is oriented toward logic and deals with one thing after the other. The female side in us is able to do many things at once. Men are neither right-brain amputated, nor are women left-brain amputated. Thus, another argument for discrimination against men is debunked as total nonsense.

OK, excursion over; back to the Sun. Its energy gives us the strength to live, to melt the ice and to let life blossom.

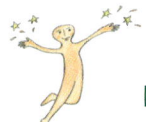

Dad, I'm coming home

"Father Sun,
as a part of you,
you are fully in me
and live through me."

Does this statement generate stress when you feel it, say it or test it with the arm-length test? If so, balance the stress.

Can you now feel the rhythm of the Great Father, his heart, his warmth and love, and become one with him again?

Now we proceed to the infinite reaches of the universe. One of the ancient hermetic laws states: "As above, so below." Thus, our body, too, is just a reflection of the whole universe.

Each of our organs has its own rhythm. We all know the heart rhythm, the pulse and the rhythm of our breath. As you already know, even our skull has its own rhythm.

And for the eternal skeptics who can't imagine the skull breathing—though I doubt they made it this far in our course—another self-experiment: Take a belt and put it around your head. Tighten it as much as possible, and now have fun! If afterward, you still doubt the individual breath and rhythm of your skull, I'm sorry, but I can't help you anymore. Blocking the cranial rhythm is one of the most horrible torture methods; it corresponds to the eternal skeptics' mode of life, those who love to block the natural development of things, to heighten the pressure, and by doing this, draw attention to themselves.

Back to the rhythms of the body: The liver, too, has its own rhythm. With this, I don't mean drinking beer every 24 hours, but the vibration in which it moves or breathes. The kidneys also have their own breath, like any other organ in our wonderful body.

The world is sound, and our body a symphony.

The same is true for the universe with all its planets, stars and galaxies, each sounding, vibrating and breathing differently. Our body is a reflection of this. We are divine music.

Therapists, for example, use tuning forks attuned to the frequencies of the planets, and thus are able to achieve some astounding miracles with them.

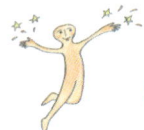

Sounds of the Worlds, I'm coming home

"Universe,
as a part of you,
you are fully in me
and live through me."

Does this statement generate stress when you feel it, say it or test it with the arm-length test? If so, balance the stress.

Imagine you are the universe, and your organs the galaxies—each one vibrating in its own original sound. You are music, the music of the spheres. This is very beneficial and healing.

The only thing left now is the absolute, the non-dual, God, the Source itself. Don't be shy and get in touch directly with God, the Source—God doesn't need a translator or a representative on Earth who can bring you his or her messages—God is inside each and everyone of us.

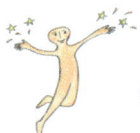

God, Source, I'm coming home

"God,
as a part of you,
you are fully in me
and live through me."

Does this statement generate stress when you feel it, say it or test it with the arm-length test? If so, balance the stress.

I am one with all that is.

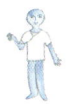 Once you have connected yourself again with your Great Mother, the Father, the Universe and the Source, your gifts will be ready for you to enjoy:

Imagine again doing a cartwheel on the balancing beam. Any changes? Are you still falling down? Are you now landing on your feet? Whether you want to try a real balancing beam and do a reality check, I leave this to your own feeling and perception of your body and your responsibility. The fact that something can be imagined doesn't necessarily mean it can be done right away. Many muscle groups have become atrophied and tendons shortened, because they haven't been used. But if you keep practicing, you can do it.

It's not just the balance that changes. Many more gifts will be given to you, you're connected with everything again—a connection that the ancient cultures of humanity have always cherished, and that has given them their inner and energetic stability—the foundation of trust in life.

Your teeth will also change. They want to get back to their original place. Their movement no longer generates stress. They can move freely again, and if you have braces, the time you'll need to wear them will be significantly less.

Now move your teeth again back and forth with your tongue and imagine again that they can turn a little. Using the arm-length test, find out if there's still stress. If so, treat the residual stress with *The Complete Healing System.*

Also note: What has changed in your brain? Which brainwave frequencies love the connection to the Earth, Sun, Sounds of the Worlds and God?

29.

YOUR PERSONAL INDEPENDENCE DAY

 Now go and be your own healer and celebrate your personal Independence Day!

With this course in healing, you have completed the first step of your education as a healer.

Enjoy your new freedom and begin your journey of discovery.

And this is precisely the fascinating aspect for everyone who works professionally with *innerwise*—discovering something new with each encounter, learning new things and being allowed to grow. *innerwise* is magic.

I have one more parameter to test how grown-up you are:

Social maturity

Do you behave like a child, or like a grown-up? Our social maturity is not always the same. Oftentimes it depends on the situation. When we visit our parents, we turn into children again; at work, we're playing another role with a different social maturity. Grown-ups sometimes act like children, and children prematurely like grown-ups.

You can test your maturity in years, and it should be similar in all areas of your life, let's say plus or minus five years. And it should correspond to your true age.

Please also test this question when you're visiting your parents, at school, at work, or in the presence of your partner. We're able to take on many different roles.

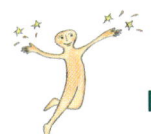

My social maturity is:

When I am with my partner:	___ years
When I am alone:	___ years
When I visit my parents:	___ years
When I am at work:	___ years
When I am with my children:	___ years
If I were on stage:	___ years

And here an overview of the test questions for you:

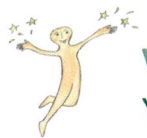

Video clip 16 Daily checkup
Your daily health check

	Optimal value	
Initial state	Arms equally long; balance	
Reaction to stress "No"	Arms differ in length	
I am I	Yes	
Number of energy fields	1	

 You can test the list from top to bottom and immediately work on the areas where you have stress.

However, it's easier and faster if you don't test one by one; instead, test intuitively, and immediately treat any stress you find. Usually this cuts the amount of work in half, since the issues depend on one another.

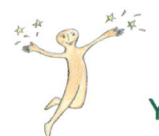

Your weekly health check

	Optimal value	
Life energy	100%	
Biological age	Younger than your actual age	
Actual creative potential	At least 30%	
Social maturity	Age-appropriate	
Heart	Stress-free	
Breathing	Stress-free	
Kidneys	Stress-free	
Liver, gallbladder	Stress-free	
Pancreas	Stress-free	
Nervous system: brain, spinal cord, nerves	Stress-free	
Autonomic nervous system: pelvic plexus, solar plexus, cervical plexus	Stress-free	
Yes to change	Stress-free	
Yes to love	Stress-free	
Yes to the body	Stress-free	
Yes to life	Stress-free	
Yes to honesty	Stress-free	
Yes to happiness	Stress-free	
Yes to health	Stress-free	

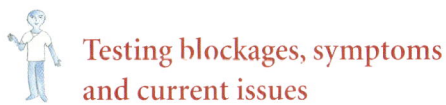

Testing blockages, symptoms and current issues

Some time ago I had rhetoric coaching because I often talk too fast, and my speech gets slurred.

When I did the arm-length test, the idea of speaking slowly and in a distinct manner generated stress in me. Within the last four hours of testing I had just introduced the rhetoric coaches to *innerwise*. So they tested me. The homework they wanted me to do generated stress, which meant that I wouldn't have done it anyway.

Then they tested me to find out where the blockages came from.

After one minute they had found the answer: In certain situations where I had to speak, my breathing was blocked because of experiences I had in my first year at school. I had adopted the thinking patterns of my teacher. Suddenly, after 38 years, all the images and feelings from that time were present again. I saw myself as a boy in that classroom where—being left handed—I was forced to change into a right-hander, and it did not feel good at all.

My rhetoric coaches drew a healing card that I virtually handed to my teacher; next, they drew a healing card for me. Now all stress was gone, my breathing opened, my pelvis got warm and my right foot started to work. And my voice was magnificently strong and deep. A man, finally!

It was a wonderful feeling, and another step on the way toward complete health.

Treating issues and symptoms

Think about the issue, and if it generates stress, clear it up.

Look at the meaning of the remedies that helped you to dissolve the stress. What did your issue stand for? Why was it still blocked? Be aware and ask questions, even if you don't get answers right away.

With a little practice, you can sense what the situation is even from a distance and work on it.

When your child is away and you sense that something is wrong, or if your child gets in touch with you to let you know that he or she needs your help, you can test whatever is necessary and send him or her the appropriate healing frequencies also from afar.

Give your child a bottle of water to hold, test the necessary healing cards until you get "no" as an answer to the question if there is anything more you can do. Then visualize the energy flowing from the healing cards into the water bottle your child is holding in his or her hand. And that is all, nothing more is needed. Now your child has the perfect remedy at his or her disposal. Next, test how long your child should take this medication, and how many times a day.

If your test shows that the child must see a doctor where he or she is, then this, too, is the right kind of help.

And remember, we're not allowed to make it "nice and easy" for other people by taking over their tasks or challenges. We are only allowed to establish flow so they can complete their tasks on their own.

30.

DECLARING LOVE TO MR. MIND, YOUR CONSCIOUS BRAIN

We're all on an extended quest. We're searching for the perfection our soul had in the beginning, in its original state, in the Garden of Eden.

We're searching for it in ourselves and in others. We find it in others when we're love-struck, and during orgasms: like a whiff, a fleeting memory of what we have once been.

In our heart, we get close to it in love, during meditation, in faith, and in moments of creativity.

Our conscious brain (the mind) is obviously not working to capacity, as it's not able to grasp more than one to five percent of what comprises our subconscious.

As long as our thoughts contain so much destructiveness, fear and negativity, it's dangerous to expect more from the conscious mind. With greater responsibility, its potential to manifest grows as well.

And more manifestation of negativity in the form of illness, aggression and destruction will inevitably lead to the self-annihilation of humanity.

When we imagine our conscious mind grasping 50 or even 70 percent of what comprises our subconscious, or—even more magnificent—the Divine, the Creative, the Source of all that is, how wonderful the lives that we manifest could be!

There existed individuals who came close to this state, or even reached it, among them Leonardo da Vinci, Plato, Aristotle,

Albert Einstein, Wolfgang Amadeus Mozart and Burkhard Heim. Since it's only in this advanced state of Being that creativity in such beauty and abundance is possible.

They are the preeminent thinkers and creators of the human race. They were capable of tapping into a greater pool of knowledge and creative power than the majority of humanity.

Beethoven saw the Ninth Symphony before his inner eye and then wrote it down after he had already gone deaf.

The arm-length test allows us to recognize the subconscious to a high extent, and to help our conscious mind and heart stay in unison. This helps us better see how we create our lives, and thus take responsibility for ourselves.

It's the end of victimhood.

We also recognize how we shape our lives with our negative thoughts and patterns, and can change it.

The more positive and clearly we think, the greater the share of the conscious mind in the subconscious and the Divine.

Enlightenment is nothing but the divine light available to us unfiltered and undiminished.

If our subconscious is an excerpt of the Divine, in return our conscious mind is an excerpt of the subconscious.

With nearly all people I've encountered so far, the share of the conscious mind in the subconscious was only one to five percent.

The fact that this is an entirely self-regulating system means that when the conscious share is small, the subconscious share in the Divine is also small.

With such limited access to all knowledge, decisions and creative power, most people have virtually no choice other than to play the role of victim in their lives.

In Canada I once met a Buddhist monk. For a long time we just looked into each other's eyes, and in this way gave each other our gifts. Even now, many years later, I can still fully feel his presence.

His conscious mind was almost equal to his subconscious. The abundance of wisdom and light shining from his eyes and his entire being enlightened everything around him, and still continues to do so.

He is a messenger of the new era, where the conscious mind and the heart create our lives in unison. When the mind coalesces with vastness and wisdom, and Mr. Mind can finally take on the role that it deserves, the dark era of humanity is over.

Presently not only the conscious mind and the subconscious show a ratio of 5 to 95 percent. The same is true for the proportion of light to darkness; trust to fear; people who create out of their own energy, to those who live on energy vampirism; creators to dependent people; visible matter to dark matter; love to the pain body; used parts of our brain to idle ones; and also the proportion of power and wealth to powerlessness and poverty here on Earth.

The opportunity for us to create a balance between all these areas is the next step of our evolution.

Then the *Homo sapiens* can become the *Homo integer*— the integrated human: the pure, decent, intact, whole, sound, honest, unblemished, unspoiled, pristine, authentic, unbroken, complete and incorruptible human.

* * *

This was our shared journey, or just the beginning of it. I was only your companion.

Now you've learned the basic ideas of *innerwise*. It's not a theoretical system; it's a living being.

An intelligent being that continuously transforms and evolves.

Oftentimes, there are people in my workshops who had dreamed the word *innerwise*, and then looked it up on the Internet, and found it. One woman in Namibia all of a sudden saw the term *innerwise* appearing on the screen of her computer.

When I began my journey in 1995, suddenly the word *innerwise* flashed before my inner eye—the connection to inner wisdom. Being able to heal oneself by reconnecting to this wisdom.

innerwise has always chosen the human beings through whom it wants to manifest itself here. Sounds like magic? Yes, *innerwise* truly IS magic, and one of the most wonderful ways to experience enlightenment here on Earth, step by step. Welcome!

Now it's time for you to read again your wishes from the second chapter, the beginning of our journey. Have they come true already? And where does your journey lead you now?

May I suggest you read the book again—one chapter per day. That had been my original idea, but who has that kind of patience the first time around?

innerwise workshops and online courses

If you like me or another *innerwise* mentor as companion, we offer a variety of workshops and online courses:

1. Yes or No—The Arm-Length Test
2. Basic workshops
3. Intensive workshops that help you work with the entire *innerwise* system
4. Practice workshops for all those interested in going deeper and developing further

I've always been a fan of "learning by doing," of short, intensive and good trainings, which allow me to then confront life and let myself be guided.

My vision is that people in all professions and areas of life will integrate energy work, and, by doing so, will make their lives, and thus the world, more beautiful and happier.

And here's one last gift for you:

I've shown you spherical vision as a way of looking at things to help you test in an objective and correct manner.

Spherical vision is one possibility. While you continue with your development, you'll discover further possibilities.

From my experience there are three levels:

I am I

Your personal point of view. That's the normal way of looking at things.
With spherical vision, we still have a chance to see things objectively or with neutrality.

I am
I am I and *I am you*.
We're capable to connect with our counterpart in such a way that we become one for the time being.

Being
All is one.
In Being, the *I am I*, and the *I am you* dissolve.

Experiencing all these levels was the greatest gift ever given to me as a human being.

innerwise—the art of flow, for living life as a naturally unfolding activity.

Here's one more of my favorite exercises:

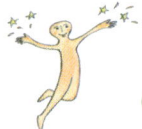

Opening our hearts to each other

Stand facing another person; if you have the courage, choose someone you don't know yet.
   Now open your heart to this person and feel how he or she opens his or her heart to you.
   After some minutes you give each other a sign and close your hearts for one another.
   What does this feel like?
   Next put your hands on each other's heart.
   Can you still keep your hearts closed off to one another?
   Sometimes one only needs a loving touch to heal.

Meditations and healing symbols

Put your hand on the symbol; close your eyes; listen and let it happen.

Then we will meet in the eternal state of simply Being.

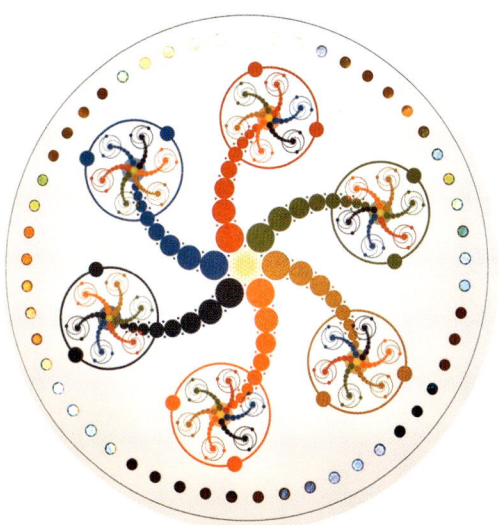

Epilog

 Hey sweetheart, as you may have noticed we didn't really have much to say in the last acts while the Doc turned into a solo entertainer. Though I've the feeling that the book is not finished yet. What do you think? Do you feel the same way?

 Yes, I feel the same, but I didn't want to impose myself just to show how smart I am.

 I feel honored that you use the word "smart" in regard to yourself.
Tell me, did the Doc even understand the quintessence of healing, the most important question?

 I don't think so. Maybe he will never understand it.

 But we can't leave the reader waiting until the Doc finally gets it.

 The Doc always says that people should be kind of disrespectful, should put everything in question and develop it further on their own. That means that we can be totally uninhibited now.
For me, the most important question is: Do people live their life purpose? Only living one's purpose nourishes people with all the energy they need to really live their lives.

I'd simply like to introduce three more parameters that the readers can test in percentages to know where they are in their lives at this point, and so that they can determine which direction is the right one, because then the percentages increase.

Finding my soul purpose in % _____

Embracing my soul purpose in % _____

Living my soul purpose in % _____

* * *

"I believe that healing through spiritual methods, in a non-material way, has a future of undreamed-of possibilities. And I believe that their range will gradually grow above and beyond what we—rightfully or not—call ›functional‹ today, and also encompass everything organic. I see the dawn of a new age shining forth before me when certain surgical interventions, such as those on internal growths or tumors, will be considered mere patchwork. We will feel absolutely horrified that our knowledge of healing methods was once so limited. Then there will hardly be any room for conventional remedies. Far be it from me to demean modern medicine and surgery in any way; on the contrary, I greatly admire both. But I've been allowed to glance at the enormous energies inherent in people, and at those of exterior sources, which, under certain circumstances, flow through them, and which I can only describe as divine—powers that can not only heal functional, but also organic disorders, which turn out to be symptoms merely accompanying emotional, mental or spiritual troubles."

—Professor Dr. med. Carl Gustav Jung, 1875–1961 (edited translation)

Biography of Uwe Albrecht

Since 1998, friends in more than 15 countries have been working under my guidance on a new healing system: *innerwise*—an energetic diagnostic, healing and development system.

With this book I would like to offer you freedom. Freedom that I've worked hard for, and that I wouldn't give up for anything in the world. The same goes for the many people who, in recent years, have learned the system with me or with other *innerwise* mentors.

It's the freedom to experience good health, happiness, creativity, freedom and abundance by accessing your inner wisdom.

Anybody can learn and use *innerwise*. My daughter Gaia was able to use it by herself when she was only two years old. One day she stood before me and said: "Daddy, you need something." Then she ordered me to lie down on the couch, crawled on top of me and tested with my arms. She chose the appropriate healing frequencies, and when everything was done, and especially when she was happy with the result, she proceeded to copy it all to an amulet so I could use it whenever necessary. I was so happy that I was given the opportunity to have this experience that it left me speechless!

I studied medicine at Humboldt University in Berlin, and became a medical doctor in 1994.

In my third academic year, I found a book on neural therapy in my mother's bookcase that she had received as a gift from a pharmaceutical representative. This book described how pain in different areas of the body had disappeared by merely injecting a local anesthetic in the gums around a particular tooth. "HEALING really does exist after all . . .," I thought. After three years of studying medicine I'd already given up hope.

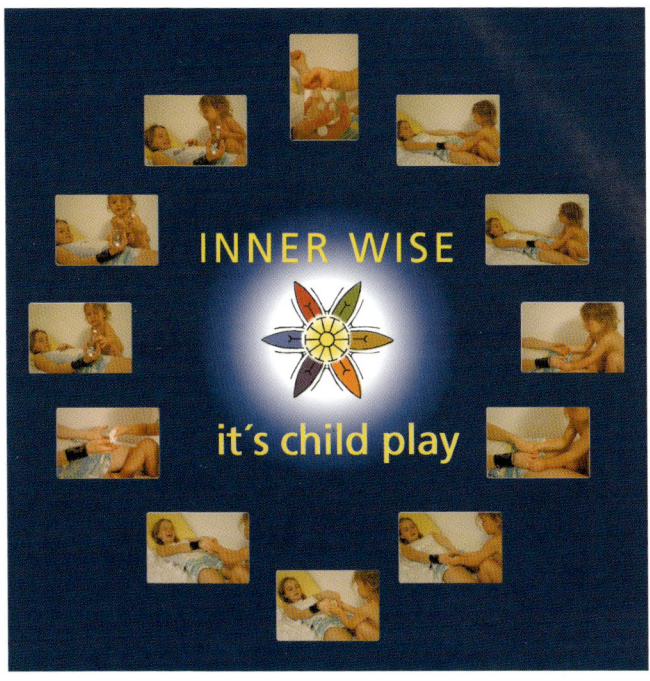

Gaia giving a treatment to her big sister

So my search began. In addition to my medical studies at the university, I started studying Traditional Chinese Medicine for several years—or to be more precise, its philosophy, pathology and medicinal herbs. I trained in neural therapy with Dr. Horst Becke, and was given the opportunity to work with Dr. Johann Abele, one of the last medical doctors who still mastered detoxifying treatments based on methods by Hufeland. The *Karl and Veronica Carstens Foundation* sponsored two clinical studies that I conducted to examine correlations between focal infections, chronic inflammations and the reflex zones in the throat and neck area; I also worked to prove the effectiveness of cupping therapy in the treatment of carpal tunnel syndrome, which otherwise often results in surgery. The studies were published internationally.

All of this was great fun, and it allowed me to meet many wonderful people including Dr. G. Draczynski, who had worked together with Professors Alfred Pischinger and Felix Perger in the seventies and who gave me precious information and texts about the ground regulation system.

Through the *Deutsche Arbeitsgemeinschaft für Herdforschung* (German Working Group on Focal Infection Research) I learned more about the implications of focal infections and their correlations within in the body. From there, my journey of discovery continued to Walter Kunnen and his son Konrad in Belgium, who became my teachers on electrosmog and geopathology. In the field of conventional medicine, I worked in different hospitals at the time. In Berlin, for example, Professor Friedrich Luft taught me to always base my therapies on the most recent studies. This became so deeply engrained in me that since then I no longer read studies and have instead set out on a journey of discovery myself.

My experiences in a rheumatic clinic focusing on autoimmune diseases (self-destructive diseases), matched exactly what I discovered later using the arm-length test: People who are ill want to be ill subconsciously. My experience working at a pain therapy clinic turned out to be the last chapter in my conventional medicine training. There, the credo was: Those who can provide healing are right. My ward physician Dr. Michael Fischer gave me the greatest amount of therapeutic freedom that one can possibly dream of. And due to the fact that at the same time I trained in physioenergetics—a kinesiological system—with Raphael von Assche, I began to use this in my work at the clinic.

This finally led to me being fired. Testing with the arms was too crazy an idea for the head of the clinical department.

What followed were trainings and profound experiences with osteopathic techniques, homeopathy, systemic constellation work and emotional therapies. For a number of years, Professor Bernd Senf worked with me using bioenergetic bodywork based on Wilhelm Reich's methods, and during one weekend I lost 1.5 diopters, which meant *no more glasses*! Another miracle!

Initially, I was supposed to take over my mother's general practice. But the thought of "processing" 60 patients a day, with only five to ten minutes time for each patient, was not possible for me anymore with the knowledge I had already acquired.

This meant that I would not have to stand on my own two feet and feed my family with my small private practice. If you're good and you can help, people will come. If you're not, they won't.

Therefore, I needed a healing system that really worked; and so I developed one myself. This system is known as ***innerwise***: healing by accessing one's inner wisdom. With this, I had found a way to combine everything I had learned so far, and to use this power to continue researching and to discover something even greater.

For me, ***innerwise*** is a living healing system that unites the best from all cultures and times. It is open, and any technique or method can be integrated. It enables us to discover individual correlations, thereby developing a new understanding of what illness is. It's both the essence and the abundance that can be applied intuitively.

It's so comprehensive and profound that it works with human beings, animals, plants, systems and projects.

My goal in working with ***innerwise*** is to eliminate blockages, to clear up old charges and programs, and in this way help to change a person's life. Then symptoms and illnesses are no longer necessary.

It's not my intention to heal people, to divest them of the developmental steps they need in order to change their lives. I simply give them back the possibility to do this themselves so they can be in the flow again and experience life as a naturally unfolding activity.

It's 2014—with the help of many dedicated people, *innerwise* has grown up and matured. There are already more than 120,000 users in some 40 countries. With the help of 40 well-trained mentors, we're ready to accept the responsibility that comes with such a gift, and make it available to as many people as possible.

Since we've been searching for the essence of healing and growth, and have gotten quite close to it, it is continually integrated into more and more areas of life:

Many people in many countries diagnose and work with themselves and others using *innerwise*:

- Medical doctors, therapists, alternative health and energy practitioners and veterinarians use *innerwise*.
- Coaches use *innerwise* to accompany businesses and projects.
- Teachers support students with *innerwise* to make learning easier.
- Geomancers use *innerwise* to clear energy fields in buildings and outdoors.
- Designers integrate *innerwise* to best adapt logos and graphics to the respective goal.
- Pharmaceutical developers create new medications using *innerwise*.
- Politicians use *innerwise* to heal historical wounds.
- Real estate agents use *innerwise* to clear up the energetic charges of buildings, which then quickly find a new owner.

And it's child's play: School children can balance themselves with *innerwise*.

Every aspect of this system is something we've experienced ourselves. As a result, some of my friends and I have gone through hell a few times and back, but have also found ourselves back on cloud nine time and again. Authenticity can't be achieved any other way. I'm grateful for all the experiences I've had in my life so far.

If I wanted to describe my path in just a few words, they would be:

- From chaos to my own identity: I am myself again, I am I.
- Trusting myself and gaining confidence
- Finally growing up and taking responsibility for my life and myself
- Reintegrating lost soul fragments
- Learning to be happy with myself
- Loving myself

As a 47-year-old, I look back at my lifework with joy, let it go and look forward to whatever life still has in store for me.

ANNEX

Emergency help in case of blockages

Easy steps you can follow in a treatment:

You're in a state of rigidity:

Intuitively draw several healing cards until the rigidity is dissolved. A maximum of eight cards may be necessary.

Your arms differ in length when first testing "yes"; they show an initial difference:

Intuitively draw some healing cards until your arms are equally long again. A maximum of five cards may be necessary.

You have a problem or a symptom:

Think of a symptom or a problem that bothers you. This will result in a difference in arm length.
Now, intuitively draw healing cards until the difference is gone. A maximum of ten cards may be necessary.

Your daily health check

	Optimal value	
Initial state	Arms equally long; balance	
Reaction to stress »No«	Arms differ in length	
I am I	Yes	
Number of energy fields	1	

Your weekly health check

	Optimal value	
Life energy	100%	
Biological age	Younger than your actual age	
Actual creative potential	At least 30%	
Social maturity	Age-appropriate	
Heart	Stress-free	
Breathing	Stress-free	
Kidneys	Stress-free	
Liver, gallbladder	Stress-free	
Pancreas	Stress-free	
Nervous system: brain, spinal cord, nerves	Stress-free	
Autonomic nervous system: pelvic plexus, solar plexus, cervical plexus	Stress-free	
Yes to change	Stress-free	
Yes to love	Stress-free	
Yes to the body	Stress-free	
Yes to life	Stress-free	
Yes to honesty	Stress-free	
Yes to happiness	Stress-free	
Yes to health	Stress-free	

Your success check

	Yes	No	Remedies, healing cards
I am happy.			
My profession is my calling.			
I earn enough money.			
I enjoy my success.			
I am honest with myself.			
I am honest with others.			
I like to take responsibility for tasks.			
I love my work.			
I deserve to be successful.			
I am good.			
I accomplish my tasks with a high degree of quality.			
I am competent in my area. I like to make decisions.			
I enjoy taking responsibility.			
I am open to new things.			
I am open to changes.			

Make a wish

I let go of or want to change:
1. _____
2. _____
3. _____

I want to experience:
1. _____
2. _____
3. _____

How high is your level of life energy?

What does your intuition tell you: How much life energy between 0 and 100 percent do you have right now? What's the first figure that comes to mind?

My life energy is: _____%

Calculation formular

100 − life energy = destructive energy

My destructive energy is: _____%

The moment of truth

For testing and marking

I love myself:	Yes ○	No ○
I am honest:	Yes ○	No ○
I forgive:	Yes ○	No ○
I am healthy:	Yes ○	No ○
I am happy:	Yes ○	No ○
I am beautiful:	Yes ○	No ○

The self-denial test

If you get "yes" as an answer, you should take a closer look and find solutions yourself.

I carry . . .% of my total burden for other people.
I let other people carry . . .% of my burden for me.

I allow other people to use me.	○ Yes	○ No
I use other people for myself.	○ Yes	○ No

Be a private detective and identify your troubles

Symptoms, irritations, illnesses	It's my issue Yes/No	I carry the issue for ...	The issue started (day/month/year)	It's related to ...	I am ready to let it go Yes/No	Remedy

Quit the game

Make a list of the 3 people
who draw the most energy FROM YOU:

1. _____

2. _____

3. _____

Make a list of the 3 people
YOU draw the most energy from:

1. _____

2. _____

3. _____

Test your biological age in years

Today my biological age is: _____ years

The "non-lovable" list

A. Facts from my past for which I can't love myself:

1. _____
2. _____
3. _____

B. Why I can't love myself now:

1. _____
2. _____
3. _____

C. Why I won't love myself in the future:

1. _____
2. _____
3. _____

And since you're at it, please write down the names of five people in your life whose lovable core you can't or don't want to see:

1. _____
2. _____
3. _____
4. _____
5. _____

Bibliography

Michel Montignac, *Eat Yourself Slim*, Erica House (1999)

James Redfield, *The Celestine Prophecies*, Warner Books (1993)

Ron Smothermon, *The Man-Woman Book: The Transformation of Love*, Context publications (1985)

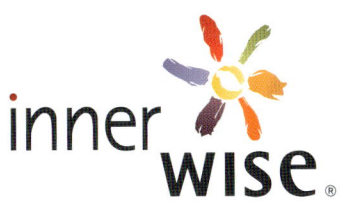
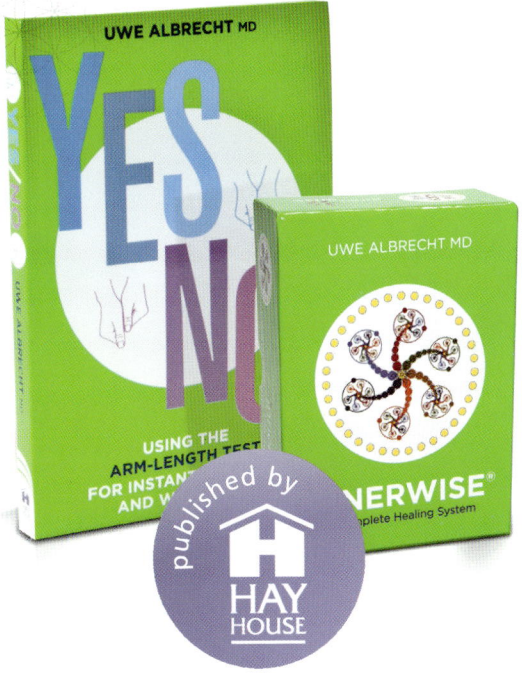

Webinare, Workshops, Therapists, Coaches and more ...

visit
www.innerwise.com • www.innerwise.us

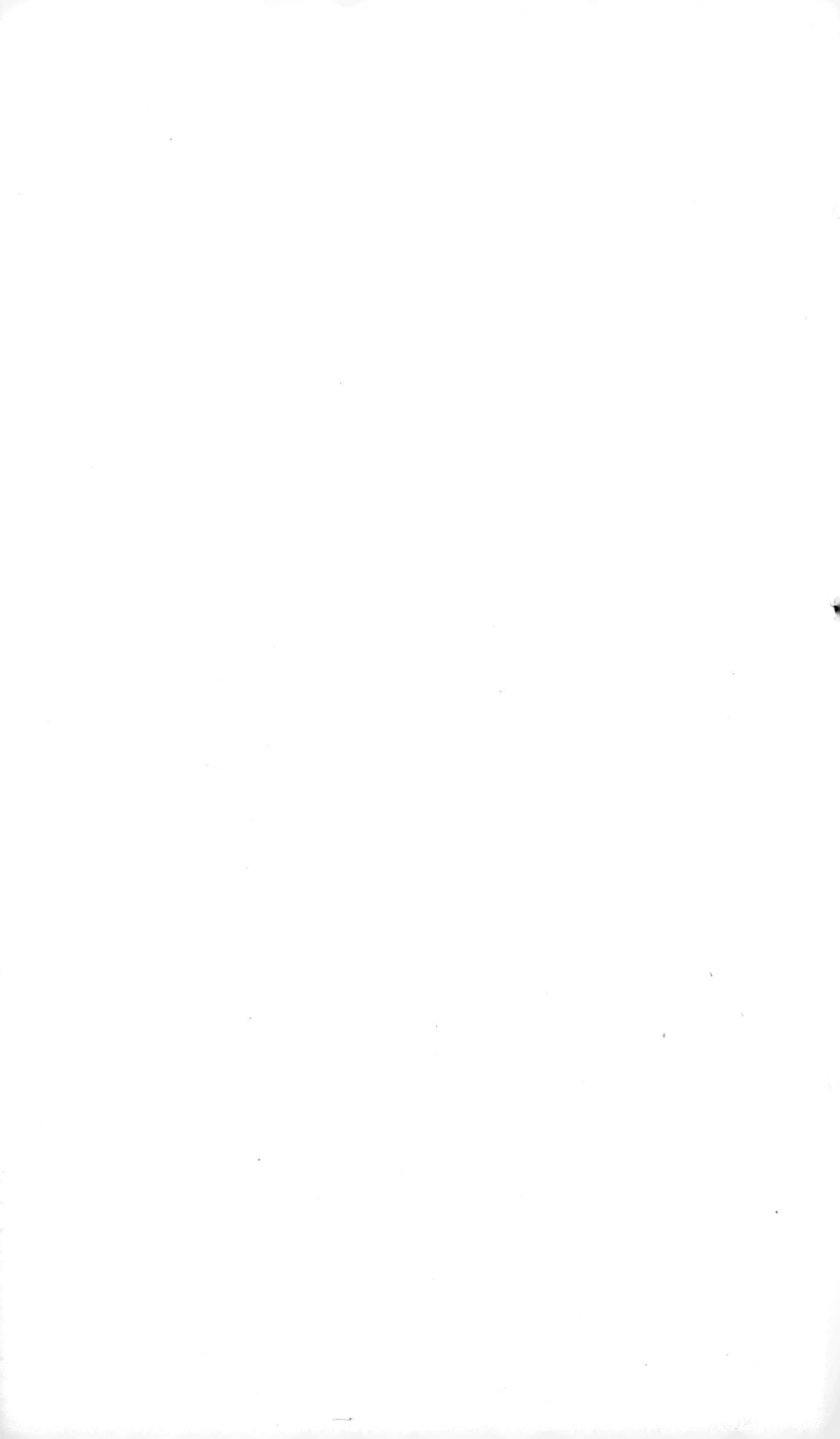